Teen Health Series

Pregnancy Information For Teens, Third Edition

Pregnancy Information For Teens, Third Edition

Health Tips About Teen Pregnancy And Teen Parenting

Including Facts About Prenatal Care, Pregnancy Complications,
Labor And Delivery, Postpartum Care, Pregnancy-Related
Lifestyle Concerns, The Emotional And Legal Issues
Of Teen Parenting, And More

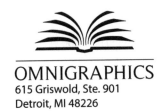

OMNIGRAPHICS
615 Griswold, Ste. 901
Detroit, MI 48226

Bibliographic Note
Because this page cannot legibly accommodate all the copyright notices, the Bibliographic Note portion of the Preface constitutes an extension of the copyright notice.

* * *

Omnigraphics
a part of Relevant Information
Keith Jones, *Managing Editor*

* * *

Copyright © 2017 Omnigraphics
ISBN 978-0-7808-1557-5
E-ISBN 978-0-7808-1558-2

Library of Congress Cataloging-in-Publication Data

Names: Omnigraphics, Inc., issuing body.

Title: Pregnancy information for teens: health tips about teen pregnancy and teen parenting including facts about prenatal care, pregnancy complications, labor and delivery, postpartum care, pregnancy-related lifestyle concerns, the emotional and legal issues of teen parenting, and more.

Description: Third edition. | Detroit, MI: Omnigraphics, [2017] | Series: Teen health series | Audience: Grade 9 to 12. | Includes bibliographical references and index.

Identifiers: LCCN 2017007851 (print) | LCCN 2017008563 (ebook) | ISBN 9780780815575 (hardcover: alk. paper) | ISBN 9780780815582 (ebook) | ISBN 9780780815582 (eBook)

Subjects: LCSH: Teenage parents. | Teenage pregnancy.

Classification: LCC HQ759.64 .P72 2017 (print) | LCC HQ759.64 (ebook) | DDC 618.200835--dc23

LC record available at https://lccn.loc.gov/2017007851

Table Of Contents

Part Four: High-Risk Pregnancies And Pregnancy Complications

Part Five: Childbirth

Part Six: Your Newborn

Part Seven: Teen Parenting Problems And Solutions

Part Eight: If You Need More Information

Preface

About This Book

According to recent data from the Centers for Disease Control and Prevention (CDC), the U.S. teenage birth rate reached a historic low in 2015, at 22.3 births per 1,000 women aged 15–19. Despite this encouraging news, the U.S. teenage birth rate retained its distinction of being the highest among industrialized countries, emphasizing the nation's need for continued efforts at helping young women avoid unplanned pregnancies.

Teenage pregnancy is associated with diverse risks. Teenage mothers have a higher risk of preterm labor and delivery, anemia, preeclampsia, and other pregnancy complications. Babies born to teenage mothers have higher risks for low birthweight, serious health problems, and even death. Some pregnant teens may lack access to proper nutrition or may participate in risky activities, such as smoking, drinking alcohol, and taking drugs, which can have a negative effect on maternal and fetal health. In addition to such physical concerns, teenage mothers— and fathers—face other social and emotional risks, including negotiating relationships with each other and with their parents. Furthermore, they are less likely than their peers to complete their education and find well-paying jobs.

Pregnancy Information For Teens, Third Edition, discusses the bewildering array of choices to be made and the obstacles to be overcome when a young woman faces an unplanned pregnancy. It includes facts about abortion, adoption, prenatal care, nutrition, fetal development, and preparing for labor and delivery. For teens choosing to parent their infants, it offers information on how to care for a newborn, locate and pay for child care, and receive child support. It discusses the importance of completing an education and describes the public assistance programs that are available, including assistance with health insurance and living arrangements. An end section provides information about sources of help and directories of additional resources.

How To Use This Book

This book is divided into parts and chapters. Parts focus on broad areas of interest; chapters are devoted to single topics within a part.

Part One: Understanding The Problem Of Teen Pregnancy discusses the serious consequences teen pregnancy has on the mother, the child, and on society. It also presents information on pregnancy prevention, and how parents can help by talking with their child about relationships and pregnancy prevention. There is also a chapter on teen pregnancy and the media that explores the impact various forms of media can have on teens' perceptions of pregnancy and parenting.

Part Two: If You Think You're Pregnant provides information on the signs and symptoms of pregnancy and facts about pregnancy tests. After a pregnancy is confirmed, pregnant teens must make a difficult choice—abortion, adoption, or parenting. Individual chapters within this part discuss each of these alternatives.

Part Three: Staying Healthy During Your Pregnancy talks about what a pregnant teen must do— and not do—in order to have a healthy pregnancy. It includes information on prenatal care, tests and procedures, sleep, nutrition, and exercise. It also explains why alcohol, tobacco, illegal drugs, and some other substances must be avoided during pregnancy.

Part Four: High-Risk Pregnancies And Pregnancy Complications discusses various conditions that may be present before pregnancy that increase the risk of complications, such as asthma and diabetes. It also discusses conditions that can arise during pregnancy, such as gestational diabetes and preeclampsia.

Part Five: Childbirth describes the many ways to prepare for childbirth, such as birthing classes, birth plans, and choosing a birth location. It also presents information on labor, birth, having a doula, and recovery.

Part Six: Your Newborn gives teen mothers important information about what happens during a newborn's first hours of life, including health assessments and screening tests. It also answers questions about breastfeeding and gives tips on taking care of a baby at home.

Part Seven: Teen Parenting Problems And Solutions discusses the many unique challenges teen parents face, including child care options, finding a place to live, and finishing school. Important facts about child custody, child care, and health insurance are presented along with public assistance options for teen parents, including supplemental nutrition and vaccine programs. Finally, there is a chapter about the rights and responsibilities of teen fathers.

Part Eight: If You Need More Information includes directories of teen pregnancy resources, assistance for low-income pregnant women, and education resources for teen parents.

Bibliographic Note

This volume contains documents and excerpts from publications issued by the following U.S. government agencies: Administration for Children and Families (ACF); Centers for Disease Control and Prevention (CDC); Centers for Medicare and Medicaid Services (CMS); Child Welfare Information Gateway; *Eunice Kennedy Shriver* National Institute of Child Health and Human Development (NICHD); Food and Nutrition Service (FNS); Genetics Home Reference (GHR); National Guideline Clearinghouse (NGC); National Institute of Diabetes and Digestive and Kidney Diseases (NIDDK); Office of Adolescent Health (OAH); Office on Women's Health (OWH); USA.gov; U.S. Consumer Product Safety Commission (CPSC); U.S. Department of Health and Human Services (HHS); U.S. Department of Housing and Urban Development (HUD); U.S. Environmental Protection Agency (EPA); U.S. Food and Drug Administration (FDA); and U.S. National Institutes of Health (NIH).

In addition, this volume contains copyrighted documents from the following organizations: American Pregnancy Association; National Association of Child Care Resource & Referral Agencies (NACCRRA); The Nemours Foundation; and Planned Parenthood Federation of America Inc.

It may also contain original material produced by Omnigraphics and reviewed by medical consultants.

The photograph on the front cover is © monkeybusinessimages/iStock.

Medical Review

Omnigraphics contracts with a team of qualified, senior medical professionals who serve as medical consultants for the *Teen Health Series*. As necessary, medical consultants review reprinted and originally written material for currency and accuracy. Citations including the phrase, Reviewed (month, year)" indicate material reviewed by this team. Medical consultation services are provided to the *Teen Health Series* editors by:

Dr. Vijayalakshmi, MBBS, DGO, MD
Dr. Senthil Selvan, MBBS, DCH, MD
Dr. K. Sivanandham, MBBS, DCH, MS (Research), PhD

About The *Teen Health Series*

At the request of librarians serving today's young adults, the *Teen Health Series* was developed as a specially focused set of volumes within Omnigraphics' *Health Reference Series*. Each volume deals comprehensively with a topic selected according to the needs and interests of people in middle school and high school. Teens seeking preventive guidance, information about disease warning signs, medical statistics, and risk factors for health problems will find answers to their questions in the *Teen Health Series*. The *Series*, however, is not intended to serve as a tool for diagnosing illness, in prescribing treatments, or as a substitute for the physician/patient relationship. All people concerned about medical symptoms or the possibility of disease are encouraged to seek professional care from an appropriate healthcare provider.

If there is a topic you would like to see addressed in a future volume of the *Teen Health Series*, please write to:

Editor
Teen Health Series
Omnigraphics
615 Griswold, Ste. 901
Detroit, MI 48226

A Note About Spelling And Style

Teen Health Series editors use *Stedman's Medical Dictionary* as an authority for questions related to the spelling of medical terms and the *Chicago Manual of Style* for questions related to grammatical structures, punctuation, and other editorial concerns. Consistent adherence is not always possible, however, because the individual volumes within the *Series* include many documents from a wide variety of different producers and copyright holders, and the editor's primary goal is to present material from each source as accurately as is possible following the terms specified by each document's producer. This sometimes means that information in different chapters or sections may follow other guidelines and alternate spelling authorities.

Part One
Understanding The Problem Of Teen Pregnancy

Chapter 1
The Risks Of Teenage Pregnancy

Parenting at any age can be challenging, but it can be particularly difficult for adolescent parents. In 2015, just over 229,000 babies were born to teen girls between the ages of 15 and 19. Childbearing during adolescence negatively affects the parents, their children, and society. Compared with their peers who delay childbearing, teen girls who have babies are:

- Less likely to finish high school;

- More likely to rely on public assistance;

- More likely to be poor as adults; and

- More likely to have children who have poorer educational, behavioral, and health outcomes over the course of their lives than do kids born to older parents.

Teen childbearing costs U.S. taxpayers billions of dollars due to lost tax revenue, increased public assistance payments, and greater expenditures for public healthcare, foster care, and criminal justice services.

The good news is that teen birth rates in the United States have declined almost continuously since the early 1990s—including an eight percent drop from 2014 to 2015—further decreasing from 2014's historic lows. Between 1991 and 2015, the teen birth rate decreased by more than half in the United States (from 61.8 to 22.3 per 1,000 teens). Despite this decline, the U.S. teen birth rate is still higher than that of many other developed countries, including Canada and the United Kingdom.

About This Chapter: This chapter includes text excerpted from "Teen Pregnancy And Childbearing," Office of Adolescent Health (OAH), U.S. Department of Health and Human Services (HHS), March 11, 2017.

Recent studies have explored strategies to reduce teen childbearing and its associated negative outcomes for parents, children, and society. For example, results from economic analyses suggest that implementing evidence-based teen pregnancy prevention programs, expanding access to Medicaid family planning services, and utilizing mass media campaigns to promote safe sex may reduce teen pregnancy and save taxpayer dollars. Additionally, the Pregnancy Assistance Fund (PAF) initiative of the Office of Adolescent Health (OAH) was set up to help pregnant and parenting teens receive the education, healthcare, parenting skills, and additional supports that they need. This help, in turn, may improve the likelihood of success in adulthood for these young parents, and reduce the probability that they will have or father other children as teens and that their children will grow up to become teen parents.

Teen Pregnancy Prevention Program

OAH leads a new evidence-based initiative to reduce teen pregnancy, human immunodeficiency virus (HIV) and other sexually transmitted diseases (STDs), and risky sexual behavior among adolescents. Funding from the Teen Pregnancy Prevention Program (TPP) supports competitive grants to public and private entities to fund medically accurate and age-appropriate programs that reduce teen pregnancy and the federal costs associated with administration and evaluation. A key component underlying OAH's grant programs is an independent, systematic review of the evidence base on programs to reduce teen pregnancy, STDs, and associated sexual risk behaviors. The review identifies, assesses, and rates the rigor of program evaluation studies and describes the strength of evidence supporting different program models. Findings are used to identify program models that meet the criteria for the U.S. Department of Health and Human Services (HHS) Teen Pregnancy Prevention Evidence Review. Identifying these evidence-based programs allows for replication and testing of the programs in different settings or with different populations to learn more about the programs' effectiveness, and to undertake and test new, innovative programs or to test significant adaptations to an evidence-based program.

The OAH administers a two-tiered TPP grant program and works in concert with closely aligned programs supported by other federal agencies.

1. **Replication of Evidence-Based Programs:** OAH funds replications of 23 of the program models from the HHS Teen Pregnancy Prevention Evidence Review through 75 different grantees, with some grantees replicating more than one model. Funded organizations selected the program model or models to replicate based on their communities' needs. The evaluation of these replications will contribute additional knowledge about these program models.

2. **Research and Demonstration Projects:** To develop and test additional models and innovative strategies to prevent teen pregnancy, OAH funds 19 TPP research and demonstrations programs, and the Administration on Children and Families (ACF) funds an additional 13 innovative strategy projects targeting vulnerable populations, such as youth in foster care and homeless youth. OAH also provides funds for the Centers for Disease Control and Prevention (CDC) to implement and test community-wide approaches to teen pregnancy prevention, focusing on eight communities with very high teen birth rates. These federal agencies collaborate to provide technical assistance, information exchange, and reporting among grantees.

In addition, the Affordable Care Act provides funding to replicate evidence-based teen pregnancy prevention program models through the Personal Responsibility Education Program (PREP), administered by the Family Youth Service Bureau (FYSB) within ACF.

The ACF/FYSB prevention programs include several distinct components,

- *formula grants* to states to either replicate evidence-based effective programs or to substantially incorporate elements of effective prevention programs while including three of six adult preparation subjects mandated by Congress;
- *competitive PREP Innovative Strategies (PREIS) cooperative agreement grants,* which were issued in conjunction with the OAH research and demonstration grants;
- discretionary 3-year grants based on unexpended allotments from states and Territories that did not apply for PREP in FY 2011 and 2012;
- *grants provided for Indian Tribes and Tribal organizations*; and
- a competitive abstinence program.

(Source:"Pregnancy Prevention," Youth.gov.)

Characteristics Associated With Adolescent Childbearing

Numerous individual, family, and community characteristics have been linked to adolescent childbearing. For example, adolescents who are enrolled in school and engaged in learning (including participating in after-school activities, having positive attitudes toward school, and performing well educationally) are less likely than are other adolescents to have or to father a baby. At the family level, adolescents with mothers who gave birth as teens and/or whose mothers have only a high school degree are more likely to have a baby before age 20 than are teens whose mothers were older at their birth or who attended at least some college. In addition, having lived with both biological parents at age 14 is associated with a lower risk of a teen birth. At the community level, adolescents who live in wealthier neighborhoods with strong levels of employment are less likely to have or to father a baby than are adolescents in neighborhoods in which income and employment opportunities are more limited.

Negative Impacts Of Teen Childbearing

Teen childbearing is associated with negative consequences for the adolescent parents, their children, and society.

Children born to adolescents face particular challenges—they are more likely to have poorer educational, behavioral, and health outcomes throughout their lives, compared with children born to older parents.

Moreover, teen childbearing costs U.S. taxpayers between $9.4 and $28 billion a year through public assistance payments, lost tax revenue, and greater expenditures for public healthcare, foster care, and criminal justice services.

Chapter 2
Recent Teen Pregnancy Statistics

Pregnancy Rates In The United States

The 2015 number of U.S. births was 3,977,745, down slightly (less than 1%) from 2014. The general fertility rate was 62.5 births per 1,000 women aged 15–44, down less than 1 percent from 2014. The birth rate for teenagers aged 15–19 decreased 8 percent in 2015 to 22.3 births per 1,000 women, another historic low for the country; rates decreased for both younger and older teenagers to record lows. The birth rate for women in their early 20s declined to 76.9 births per 1,000 women, another record low. The nonmarital birth rate declined 1 percent in 2015, to 43.5 births per 1,000 unmarried women aged 15–44. The Cesarean delivery rate declined for the third year in a row to 32 percent, and the low-risk Cesarean delivery rate declined again to 25.7 percent in 2015. The low birthweight rate was up in 2015 to 8.07 percent.

> The preterm birth rate rose slightly to 9.63% from 2014 to 2015.
>
> *(Source: Births In The United States, 2015, Centers for Disease Control and Prevention (CDC).)*

Births And Birth Rates

- The **general fertility rate** (GFR) for the United States also decreased less than 1 percent in 2015, to 62.5 births per 1,000 women aged 15–44, from 62.9 in 2014. This decline follows an increase in the rate from 2013 to 2014, the first increase since 2007.

About This Chapter: Text beginning with the heading "Pregnancy Rates In The United States" is excerpted from "National Vital Statistics Reports," Centers for Disease Control and Prevention (CDC), June 2, 2016; Text beginning with the heading "Socioeconomic Disparities" is excerpted from "Social Determinants And Eliminating Disparities In Teen Pregnancy," Centers for Disease Control and Prevention (CDC), August 8, 2016.

- The **birth rate for teenagers** in 2015 was 22.3 births per 1,000 women aged 15–19— yet another historic low for the country. The rate was down 8 percent from 2014 (24.2) and has declined more than 46 percent since 2007. Since the most recent peak in 1991 (61.8), the rate has declined a total of 64 percent. In 2015, the number of births to women aged 15–19 was 229,888, down 8 percent from 2014 and 48 percent from 2007 (444,899).

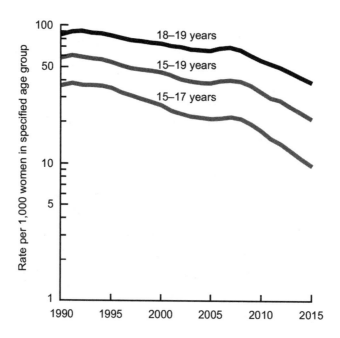

Figure 2.1. Birth Rates For Women Aged 15–19

- In 2015, the birth rates for teenagers aged 15–17 and 18–19 fell 9 percent and 7 percent, respectively, to 9.9 and 40.7 births per 1,000 women. These rates were yet another record low for both groups, from 10.9 and 43.8 in 2014. Since 2007, the rate for teenagers aged 15–17 has dropped 54 percent, and the rate for those aged 18–19 has dropped 43 percent. The number of births for teenagers aged 15–17 declined 8 percent from 2014 to 2015, and births to those aged 18–19 declined 7 percent.

- The birth rate for females aged 10–14 was 0.2 births per 1,000 in 2015, declining from 2014 (0.3), to a new historic low for the country. The number of births to mothers in this age group declined 10 percent in 2015, to 2,503 births.

Table 2.1. Births And Birth Rates, By Age Of Mother

Age Of Mother	2015		2014		Percent Change
	Number	Rate	Number	Rate	2014–2015
10–14	2,503	0.2	2,769	0.3	–33
15–19	229,888	22.3	249,078	24.2	–8
• 15–17	• 61,223	• 9.9	• 66,791	• 10.9	• –9
• 18–19	• 168,665	• 40.7	• 182,287	• 43.8	• –7

- The **birth rate for unmarried women** in 2015 was 43.5 births per 1,000 unmarried women aged 15–44, down 1% from 2014 (43.9) and marking the seventh consecutive year of decline since the all-time peak in 2007 and 2008 (51.8).

  - In 2015, the number of births to unmarried women was 1,600,208, a less than 1 percent (0.3%) decline from 2014 (1,604,870). The 2015 number of nonmarital births was 7 percent lower than the 2008 peak (1,726,566).

Socioeconomic Disparities

Socioeconomic conditions in communities and families may contribute to high teen birth rates. Examples of these factors include—

- Low education and low income levels of a teen's family.

- Few opportunities in a teen's community for positive youth involvement.

- Neighborhood racial segregation.

- Neighborhood physical disorder (graffiti, abandoned vehicles, litter, alcohol containers, cigarette butts, glass on the ground).

- Neighborhood-level income inequality.

- Teens in child welfare systems are at increased risk of teen pregnancy and birth than other groups. For example, young women living in foster care are more than twice as likely to become pregnant than those not in foster care.

Taking Action To Eliminate Disparities And Address Social Determinants Of Teen Pregnancy

Eliminating disparities in teen pregnancy and birth rates would—

- Help achieve health equity.

- Improve the life opportunities and health outcomes of young people.

- Reduce the economic costs of teen childbearing.

Efforts that focus on social determinants of health in teen pregnancy prevention efforts, particularly at the community level, play a critical role in addressing racial/ethnic and geographical disparities observed in teen births in the United States.

Chapter 3

When Pregnancy Is A Result Of Abuse

Domestic violence is when one person in a relationship purposely hurts another person physically or emotionally. Domestic violence is also called intimate partner violence because it often is caused by a husband, ex-husband, boyfriend, or ex-boyfriend. Women also can be abusers.

People of all races, education levels, and ages experience domestic abuse. In the United States, more than 5 million women are abused by an intimate partner each year.

Domestic violence includes:

- **Physical abuse** like hitting, shoving, kicking, biting, or throwing things

- **Emotional abuse** like yelling, controlling what you do, or threatening to cause serious problems for you

- **Sexual abuse** like forcing you to do something sexual you don't want to do

Adolescents with a history of physical or sexual abuse have an increased risk of teen pregnancy. In fact, when adolescents experience both sexual and physical abuse, their risk of early pregnancy is increased fourfold.

(Source: "Co-occurring Risks In Adolescence: Implications For Teen Pregnancy Prevention," Office of Adolescent Health (OAH), U.S. Department of Health and Human Services (HHS).)

About This Chapter: Text in this chapter begins with excerpts from "Violence Against Women," Office on Women's Health (OWH), U.S. Department of Health and Human Services (HHS), September 30, 2015; Text under the heading "Abuse And Pregnancy" is excerpted from "Staying Healthy And Safe," Office on Women's Health (OWH), U.S. Department of Health and Human Services (HHS), September 27, 2010. Reviewed March 2017; Text under the heading "Child Abuse And Neglect: Consequences" is excerpted from "Child Abuse And Neglect: Consequences," Centers for Disease Control and Prevention (CDC), March 28, 2016.

Here are some key points about domestic and intimate partner violence:

- **If you are in immediate danger, you can call 911.** It is possible for the police to arrest an abuser and to escort you and your children to a safe place.

- **Often, abuse starts as emotional abuse and then becomes physical later.** It's important to get help early.

- **Sometimes it is hard to know if you are being abused.** Learn more about signs of abuse (www.womenshealth.gov/violence-against-women/am-i-being-abused/index.html).

- **Your partner may try to make you feel like the abuse is your fault.** Remember that you cannot make someone mistreat you. The abuser is responsible for his or her behavior. Abuse can be a way for your partner to try to have control over you.

- **Violence can cause serious physical and emotional problems,** including depression and posttraumatic stress disorder. It's important to try to take care of your health. And if you are using drugs or alcohol to cope with abuse, get help.

- **There probably will be times when your partner is very kind.** Unfortunately, abusers often begin the mistreatment again after these periods of calm. In fact, over time, abuse often gets worse, not better. Even if your partner promises to stop the abuse, make sure to learn about hotlines and other ways to get help for abuse.

- **An abusive partner needs to get help from a mental health professional.** But even if he or she gets help, the abuse may not stop.

Being hurt by someone close to you is awful. Reach out for support from family, friends, and community organizations.

Abuse And Pregnancy

It's hard to be excited about the new life growing inside of you if you're afraid of your partner. Abuse from a partner can begin or increase during pregnancy and can harm you and your unborn baby. Women who are abused often don't get the prenatal care their babies need. Abuse from a partner also can lead to preterm birth and low birth weight babies, stillbirth and newborn death, and homicide. If you are abused, you might turn to alcohol, cigarettes, or drugs to help you cope. This can be even more harmful to you and your baby.

You may think that a new baby will change your situation for the better. But the cycle of abuse is complex, and a baby introduces new stress to people and relationships. Now is a good time to think about your safety and the safety and wellbeing of your baby. About 50 percent of men who abuse their wives also abuse their children. Think about the home environment you want for your baby. Studies show that children who witness or experience violence at home may have long-term physical, emotional, and social problems. They are also more likely to experience or commit violence themselves in the future.

Prevalence Of Child Abuse

- 1 in 4 children suffer abuse.
- An estimated 702,000 children were confirmed by child protective services as being victims of abuse and neglect in 2014.
- At least one in four children have experienced child neglect or abuse (including physical, emotional, and sexual) at some point in their lives, and one in seven children experienced abuse or neglect in the last year.

(Source: "Child Abuse And Neglect: Consequences," Centers for Disease Control and Prevention (CDC).)

Prenatal exams offer a good chance to reach out for help. It's possible to take control and leave an abusive partner. But for your and your baby's safety, talk to your doctor first. Let motherhood prompt you to take action now.

If you're a victim of abuse or violence at the hands of someone you know or love, or you are recovering from an assault by a stranger, you and your baby can get immediate help and support.

- The National Domestic Violence Hotline can be reached 24 hours a day, 7 days a week at 800-799-SAFE (800-799-7233) and 800-787-3224 (TTY). Spanish speakers are available. When you call, you will first hear a recording and may have to hold. Hotline staff offer crisis intervention and referrals. If requested, they connect women to shelters and can send out written information.

- The National Sexual Assault Hotline (www.rainn.org/about-national-sexual-assault-online-hotline) can be reached 24 hours a day, 7 days a week at 800-656-4673. When you call, you will hear a menu and can choose #1 to talk to a counselor. You will then be connected to a counselor in your area who can help you. You can also visit the National Sexual Assault Online Hotline.

Child Abuse And Neglect: Consequences

Child Abuse And Neglect Affect Children

- Improper brain development

- Impaired cognitive (learning ability) and socio-emotional (social and emotional) skills

- Lower language development

- Blindness, cerebral palsy from head trauma

- Higher risk for heart, lung and liver diseases, obesity, cancer, high blood pressure, and high cholesterol

- Anxiety

- Smoking, alcoholism and drug abuse

Physical

- In 2014, approximately 1,580 children died from abuse and neglect across the country—a rate of 2.13 deaths per 100,000 children.

- Abuse and neglect during infancy or early childhood can cause regions of the brain to form and function improperly with long-term consequences on cognitive and language abilities, socioemotional development, and mental health. For example, the stress of chronic abuse may cause a "hyperarousal" response in certain areas of the brain, which may result in hyperactivity and sleep disturbances.

- Children may experience severe or fatal head trauma as a result of abuse. Nonfatal consequences of abusive head trauma include varying degrees of visual impairment (e.g., blindness), motor impairment (e.g., cerebral palsy) and cognitive impairments.

- Children who experience abuse and neglect are also at increased risk for adverse health effects and certain chronic diseases as adults, including heart disease, cancer, chronic lung disease, liver disease, obesity, high blood pressure, high cholesterol, and high levels of C-reactive protein.

Behavioral

- Children who experience abuse and neglect are at increased risk for smoking, alcoholism, and drug abuse as adults, as well as engaging in high-risk sexual behaviors.

- Those with a history of child abuse and neglect are 1.5 times more likely to use illicit drugs, especially marijuana, in middle adulthood.

- Studies have found abused and neglected children to be at least 25 percent more likely to experience problems such as delinquency, teen pregnancy, and low academic achievement. Similarly, a longitudinal study found that physically abused children were at greater risk of being arrested as juveniles, being a teen parent, and less likely to graduate high school.

- A National Institute of Justice (NIJ) study indicated that being abused or neglected as a child increased the likelihood of arrest as a juvenile by 59 percent. Abuse and neglect also increased the likelihood of adult criminal behavior by 28 percent and violent crime by 30 percent.

- Child abuse and neglect can have a negative effect on the ability of both men and women to establish and maintain healthy intimate relationships in adulthood.

Chapter 4
Preventing Teen Pregnancy

Teen childbearing can carry health, economic, and social costs for mothers and their children. Teen births in the United States have declined, but still more than 273,000 infants were born to teens ages 15 to 19 in 2013. The good news is that more teens are waiting to have sex, and for sexually active teens, nearly 90 percent used birth control the last time they had sex.

- About 43 percent of teens ages 15 to 19 have ever had sex.
- More than 4 in 5 (86%) used birth control the last time they had sex.
- Less than 5 percent of teens on birth control used the most effective types.

However, teens most often use condoms and birth control pills, which are less effective at preventing pregnancy when not used consistently and correctly. Intrauterine devices (IUDs) and implants, known as Long-Acting Reversible Contraception (LARC), are the most effective types of birth control for teens. LARC is safe to use, does not require taking a pill each day or doing something each time before having sex, and can prevent pregnancy for 3 to 10 years, depending on the method. Less than 1 percent of LARC users would become pregnant during the first year of use.

About This Chapter: Text in this chapter begins with excerpts from "Preventing Teen Pregnancy," Centers for Disease Control and Prevention (CDC), April 7, 2015; Text under the heading "CDC Priority: Reducing Teen Pregnancy And Promoting Health Equity Among Youth" is excerpted from "Social Determinants And Eliminating Disparities In Teen Pregnancy," Centers for Disease Control and Prevention (CDC), August 8, 2016; Text beginning with the heading "Strategies And Approaches For Preventing Teen Pregnancy" is excerpted from "Teen Pregnancy And Childbearing," Office of Adolescent Health (OAH), U.S. Department of Health and Human Services (HHS), March 11, 2017.

Doctors, nurses, and other healthcare providers can:

- Encourage teens not to have sex.

- Recognize LARC as a safe and effective choice of birth control for teens.

- Offer a broad range of birth control options to teens, including LARC, and discuss the pros and cons of each.

- Seek training in LARC insertion and removal, have supplies of LARC available, and explore funding options to cover costs.

- Remind teens that LARC by itself does not protect against sexually transmitted diseases and that condoms should also be used every time they have sex.

Problem

Use Of Long-Acting Reversible Contraception (LARC) Is Low

- Less than 5 percent of teens on birth control use LARC.

- Most teens use birth control pills and condoms, methods which are less effective at preventing pregnancy when not used properly.

- There are several barriers for teens who might consider LARC:

- Many teens know very little about LARC.

- Some teens mistakenly think they cannot use LARC because of their age.

- Clinics also report barriers:

- High upfront costs for supplies.

- Providers may lack awareness about the safety and effectiveness of LARC for teens.

- Providers may lack training on insertion and removal.

Providers Can Take Steps To Increase Awareness And Availability Of LARC

- Title X is a federal grant program supporting confidential family planning and related preventive services with priority for low-income clients and teens.

- Title X-funded centers have used the latest clinical guidelines on LARC, trained providers on LARC insertion and removal, and secured low- or no-cost options for birth control.

- Teen use of LARC has increased from less than 1 percent in 2005 to 7 percent in 2013.

- Other state and local programs have made similar efforts.

- More teens and young women chose LARC, resulting in fewer unplanned pregnancies.

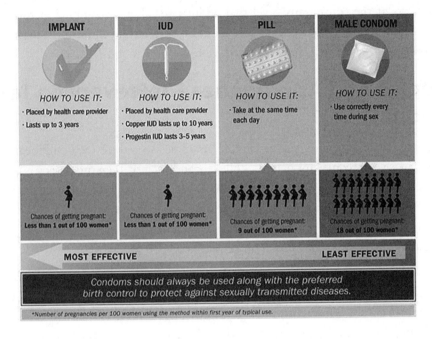

Figure 4.1. Effectiveness Of LARC

CDC Priority: Reducing Teen Pregnancy And Promoting Health Equity Among Youth

Teen pregnancy prevention is one of Centers for Disease Control and Prevention's (CDC) top seven priorities, a "winnable battle" in public health, and of paramount importance to health and quality of life for our youth. CDC supports the implementation of evidence-based teen pregnancy prevention programs that have been shown, in at least one program evaluation, to have a positive effect on preventing teen pregnancies, sexually transmitted infections, or sexual risk behaviors. Evidence-based teen pregnancy prevention programs have been identified by the U.S. Department of Health and Human Services (HHS) TPP Evidence Review, which used a systematic process for reviewing evaluation studies against a rigorous standard. Currently, the Evidence Review covers a variety of diverse programs, including sexuality education programs, youth development programs, abstinence education programs, clinic-based programs, and programs specifically designed for diverse populations and settings. In addition to evidence-based prevention programs, teens need access to youth-friendly contraceptive and reproductive health services and support from parents and other trusted adults, who can play an important role in helping teens make healthy choices about relationships, sex, and birth control. Efforts at the community level that address social and economic factors associated with teen pregnancy also play a critical role in addressing racial/ethnic and geographical disparities observed in teen births in the United States.

Strategies And Approaches For Preventing Teen Pregnancy

Efforts are currently under way to explore strategies to reduce teen childbearing and its associated negative outcomes for parents, children, and society. Teen pregnancy is estimated to cost U.S. taxpayers between $9.4 and $28 billion a year. However, research suggests that implementing evidence-based teen pregnancy prevention programs, expanding access to Medicaid family planning services, and utilizing mass media campaigns to promote safe sex may reduce teen pregnancy and lighten the burden on taxpayers.

Additionally, the Affordable Care Act, passed in 2010, aims to improve access to recommended healthcare services for the entire population, including adolescents. The law expands health insurance coverage for teens, and offers new support for preventive services, innovative models of care, and clinical training, all of which have implications for teen pregnancy in the United States.

Specific Strategies And Approaches For Adolescents

The only certain way to avoid unwanted pregnancies is to abstain from sexual intercourse. For adolescents who are sexually active, using effective contraceptives (such as condoms, birth control pills, the patch, the vaginal ring, the IUD, and/or injectable birth control methods) every time that they have sexual intercourse will reduce the risk of unwanted pregnancy. In addition to using a contraceptive method that protects against pregnancy, using condoms correctly with every sex act from start to finish will reduce the risk of human immunodeficiency virus (HIV) and other sexually transmitted diseases (STDs) for males and females.

Engaging Adolescent Males In Prevention

An estimated nine percent—or 900,000—of young men between the ages of 12 and 16 will become fathers before their 20th birthday, based on a survey conducted in 2012. Research and data collection efforts have tended to focus on female adolescents. As a result, less is known about the strategies and approaches for effectively engaging males in preventing teen pregnancies or even about their attitudes toward being a father. Clearly, the behavior of adolescent males is also central to preventing teenage pregnancy and childbearing.

> Getting young men to challenge societal presentations of masculinity can open the door to discuss teen pregnancy prevention.

Research and programs are increasing the focus on the role of males in teenage pregnancy and childrearing.

Some experts note that programs focused on responsible sexual behavior should also consider including information about how to build healthy romantic relationships overall. This would include teaching emotional and interpersonal skills and reducing gender stereotypes.

Chapter 5

Sexual Health Education: Tips For Parents

There are some tips you can follow that may help in talking with your teen about relationships and pregnancy prevention.

Start Talking

Start talking to your teen about changes to expect during puberty; your expectations for dating and contraception and condom use; how to avoid teen pregnancy, sexually transmitted diseases (STDs), and human immunodeficiency virus/acquired immunodeficiency syndrome (HIV/AIDS); and how to have healthy relationships. Talk early and often, and be ready to listen to your teen and answer questions that might come up.

Research shows that teens who talk with their parents about sex, relationships, birth control and pregnancy—

- Begin to have sex at later age.
- Use condoms and birth control more often if they do have sex.
- Have better communication with romantic partners.
- Have sex less often.

(Source: "Teen Pregnancy—Parent And Guardian Resources," Centers for Disease Control and Prevention (CDC).)

About This Chapter: This chapter includes text excerpted from "Tips For Parents," Office of Adolescent Health (OAH), U.S. Department of Health and Human Services (HHS), May 13, 2016.

Children often begin asking questions about where babies come from at a young age. These are great opportunities to lay the foundations for later talks about your expectations and values about sexual behavior and relationships. Take advantage of opportunities to have these important conversations. And if you think you waited too long, you didn't. It's never too late to begin this dialogue.

Be Clear And Specific

Be clear and specific about family values and rules about when it's okay to start dating and your expectations around dating and sexual behavior. If you have strong beliefs and values around sex and marriage, communicate those plainly. For example, if you believe people should not have sex until they are married, say that. If you think teens in high school are too young to be involved in a serious relationship, say that, and why. Or, if you think the time to have a baby is after college, say that. Same goes for using condoms or other birth control methods. Whatever your beliefs, you need to say them out loud to your son or daughter. And explain why you believe what you do.

Believe In Your Power To Affect Change

It might seem like your son or daughter is ignoring you, as if your adolescents don't want to hear what you say, or that they don't care what you think. Despite how they act, some of what you say will sink in. In survey after survey, children report that they want to talk to their parents about their sex-related questions, that it would be easier to delay sexual activity and avoid teen pregnancy if they were able to have more open, honest conversations about these topics with their parents, and that parents influence their decisions about sex more than friends do.

Be There: Monitor And Supervise

Establish rules, curfews, and expectations for behavior through family conversations. Get to know your children's friends and their families. Also, be sure to monitor what your children are reading, watching and listening to, and encourage your children to think about consequences from behaviors they may be exposed to in the media.

Discourage Early Dating

Dating during adolescence is common and can be part of healthy development. However, serious and exclusive dating relationships can lead adolescents to have sex earlier than they would have otherwise. Adolescents who have sex at an early age are more likely to engage in risky sexual behaviors and in other unsafe activities, such as substance abuse.

Ensure Your Child Has Regular Visits With A Medical Provider

Sometimes a young person will feel more comfortable asking a doctor or other medical professional specific questions about sex and reproductive health. The American Academy of Pediatrics (AAP) recommends that adolescents have private time with doctors.

Talk About Their Future

Young people who believe they have bright futures, options, and opportunities are much less likely to engage in risky sexual behavior. Encourage your children's aspirations to high levels of achievement and to participate in school and community activities (such as clubs, sports or music, etc.). Support their activities and dreams to the extent you can.

Sexual Facts

- In one study, around 70 percent of girls 15 to 19 who had sex said they wish they had waited.
- About half of teens surveyed said they never thought about what their life would be like if sex ended in pregnancy.
- You can get pregnant having sex your first time. It's possible.
- You can get pregnant having sex standing upright.
- Three out of 10 teen girls in the United States get pregnant before they turn 20.
- Most teens who become pregnant don't marry the father of their baby.
- You can get pregnant if you have sex while you are menstruating.
- One out of 4 teenage girls has a sexually transmitted disease, or STD (also known as a sexually transmitted infection, or STI).
- You cannot tell by looking at someone if they have a sexually transmitted disease, or STD (also known as a sexually transmitted infection, or STI).

(Source: "Sexual Fact Or Fiction," girlshealth.gov, Office on Women's Health (OWH).)

Chapter 6

Birth Control Methods

Birth control (contraception) is any method, medicine, or device used to prevent pregnancy. Women can choose from many different types of birth control. Some work better than others at preventing pregnancy. The type of birth control you use depends on your health, your desire to have children now or in the future, and your need to prevent sexually transmitted infections. Your doctor can help you decide which type is best for you right now.

What Is The Best Method Of Birth Control?

There is no "best" method of birth control for every woman. The birth control method that is right for you and your partner depends on many things, and may change over time.

Before choosing a birth control method, talk to your doctor or nurse about:

- whether you want to get pregnant soon, in a few years, or never

- how well each method works to prevent pregnancy

- possible side effects

- how often you have sex

- the number of sex partners you have

- your overall health

About This Chapter: This chapter includes text excerpted from "Birth Control Methods," Office on Women's Health (OWH), U.S. Department of Health and Human Services (HHS), October 15, 2015.

- how comfortable you are with using the method (For example, can you remember to take a pill every day? Will you have to ask your partner to put on a condom each time?)

Keep in mind that even the most effective birth control methods can fail. But your chances of getting pregnant are lower if you use a more effective method.

What Are The Different Types Of Birth Control?

Women can choose from many different types of birth control methods. These include, in order of most effective to least effective at preventing pregnancy:

- **Female and male sterilization** (female tubal ligation or occlusion, male vasectomy)—Birth control that prevents pregnancy for the rest of your life through surgery or a medical procedure.

- *Long-acting* **reversible contraceptives or "LARC" methods** (intrauterine devices, hormonal implants)—Birth control your doctor inserts one time and you do not have to remember to use birth control every day or month. LARCs last for 3 to 10 years, depending on the method.

- *Short-acting* **hormonal methods** (pill, mini pills, patch, shot, vaginal ring)—Birth control your doctor prescribes that you remember to take every day or month. The shot requires you to get a shot from your doctor every 3 months.

- **Barrier methods** (condoms, diaphragms, sponge, cervical cap)—Birth control you use each time you have sex.

- **Natural rhythm methods**—Not using a type of birth control but instead avoiding sex and/or using birth control only on the days when you are most fertile (most likely to get pregnant). An ovulation home test kit or a fertility monitor can help you find your most fertile days.

For Women

Table 6.1. Types Of Birth Control

Method	Number Of Pregnancies Per 100 Women Within Their First Year Of Typical Use	Side Effects And Risks*	How Often You Have To Take Or Use
Abstinence (no sexual contact)	Unknown (0 for perfect use)	No medical side effects	No action required, but it does take willpower. You may want to have a back-up birth control method, such as condoms.
Permanent sterilization surgery for women (tubal ligation, "getting your tubes tied")	Less than 1	• Possible pain during recovery (up to 2 weeks) • Bleeding or other complications from surgery • Less common risk includes ectopic (tubal) pregnancy	No action required after surgery
Permanent sterilization implant for women (Essure®)	Less than 1	• Pain during the insertion of Essure; some pain during recovery • Cramping, vaginal bleeding, back pain during recovery • Implant may move out of place • Less common but serious risk includes ectopic (tubal) pregnancy	No action required after surgery

29

Table 6.1. Continued

Method	Number Of Pregnancies Per 100 Women Within Their First Year Of Typical Use	Side Effects And Risks*	How Often You Have To Take Or Use
Implantable rod (Implanon®, Nexplanon®)	Less than 1	• Headache • Irregular periods • Weight gain • Sore breasts • Less common risk includes difficultly in removing the implant	No action required for up to 3 years before removing or replacing
Copper intrauterine device (IUD) (ParaGard®)	Less than 1	• Cramps for a few days after insertion • Missed periods, bleeding between periods, heavier periods • Less common but serious risks include pelvic inflammatory disease and the IUD being expelled from the uterus or going through the wall of the uterus.	No action required for up to 10 years before removing or replacing
Hormonal intrauterine devices (IUDs) (Liletta, Mirena®, and Skyla®)	Less than 1	• Irregular periods, lighter or missed periods • Ovarian cysts • Less common but serious risks include pelvic inflammatory disease and the IUD being expelled from the uterus or going through the wall of the uterus.	No action required for 3 to 5 years, depending on the brand, before removing or replacing

Table 6.1. Continued

Method	Number Of Pregnancies Per 100 Women Within Their First Year Of Typical Use	Side Effects And Risks*	How Often You Have To Take Or Use
Shot/injection (Depo-Provera®)	6	• Bleeding between periods, missed periods • Weight gain • Changes in mood • Sore breasts • Headaches • Bone loss with long-term use (bone loss may be reversible once you stop using this type of birth control)	Get a new shot every 3 months
Oral contraceptives, combination hormones ("the pill")	9	• Headache • Upset stomach • Sore breasts • Changes in your period • Changes in mood • Weight gain • High blood pressure • Less common but serious risks include blood clots, stroke and heart attack; the risk is higher in smokers and women older than 35	Take at the same time every day

Table 6.1. Continued

Method	Number Of Pregnancies Per 100 Women Within Their First Year Of Typical Use	Side Effects And Risks*	How Often You Have To Take Or Use
Oral contraceptives, progestin-only pill ("mini-pill")	9	• Spotting or bleeding between periods • Weight gain • Sore breasts • Headache • Nausea	Take at the same time every day
Skin patch (Xulane®)	9 May be less effective in women weighing 198 pounds or more	• Skin irritation • Upset stomach • Changes in your period • Changes in mood • Sore breasts • Headache • Weight gain • High blood pressure • Less common but serious risks include blood clots, stroke and heart attack; the risk is higher in smokers and women older than 35	Wear for 21 days, remove for 7 days, replace with a new patch

Table 6.1. Continued

Method	Number Of Pregnancies Per 100 Women Within Their First Year Of Typical Use	Side Effects And Risks*	How Often You Have To Take Or Use
Vaginal ring (NuvaRing®)	9	• Headache • Upset stomach • Sore breasts • Vaginal irritation and discharge • Changes in your period • High blood pressure • Less common but serious risks include blood clots, stroke and heart attack; the risk is higher in smokers and women older than 35	Wear for 21 days, remove for 7 days, replace with a new ring
Diaphragm with spermicide (Koromex®, Ortho-Diaphragm®)	12 If you gain or lose than 15 pounds, or have a baby, have your doctor check you to make sure the diaphragm still fits.	• Irritation • Allergic reactions • Urinary tract infection (UTI) • Vaginal infections • Rarely, toxic shock if left in for more than 24 hours • Using a spermicide often might increase your risk of getting HIV	Insert each time you have sex

Table 6.1. Continued

Method	Number Of Pregnancies Per 100 Women Within Their First Year Of Typical Use	Side Effects And Risks*	How Often You Have To Take Or Use
Sponge with spermicide (Today Sponge®)	12 (among women who have never given birth before) or 24 (among women who have given birth)	• Irritation • Allergic reactions • Rarely, toxic shock if left in for more than 24 hours • Using a spermicide often might increase your risk of getting HIV	Insert each time you have sex
Cervical cap with spermicide (FemCap®)	23	• Vaginal irritation or odor • Urinary tract infections (UTIs) • Allergic reactions • Rarely, toxic shock if left in for more than 48 hours • Using a spermicide often might increase your risk of getting HIV	Insert each time you have sex
Female condom	21	• Irritation • Condom may tear or slip out • Allergic reaction	Use each time you have sex
Natural family planning (rhythm method)	24	• Can be hard to know the days you are most fertile (when you need to avoid having sex or use back-up birth control)	Depending on method used, takes planning each month

Table 6.1. Continued

Method	Number Of Pregnancies Per 100 Women Within Their First Year Of Typical Use	Side Effects And Risks*	How Often You Have To Take Or Use
Spermicide alone	28 Works best if used along with a barrier method, such as a diaphragm	• Irritation • Allergic reactions • Urinary tract infection • Frequent use of a spermicide might increase your risk of getting HIV	Use each time you have sex

For Men

Table 6.2. Types Of Birth Control

Method	Number Of Pregnancies Per 100 Women Within Their First Year Of Typical Use	Side Effects And Risks*	How Often You Have To Take Or Use
Permanent sterilization surgery for men (vasectomy)	Less than 1	• Pain during recovery • Complications from surgery	No action required after surgery
Male condom	18	• Irritation • Condom may tear, break or slip off • Allergic reactions to latex condoms	Use each time you have sex
Withdrawal—when a man takes his penis out of a woman's vagina (or "pulls out") before he ejaculates (has an orgasm or "comes")	22	• Sperm can be released before the man pulls out, putting you at risk for pregnancy	Use each time you have sex

* These are not all of the possible side effects and risks. Talk to your doctor or nurse for more information.

Which Types Of Birth Control Can I Get Without A Prescription?

You can buy these types of birth control over-the-counter at a drugstore or supermarket:

- Male condoms

- Female condoms

- Sponges

- Spermicides

- Emergency contraception (EC) pills. Plan B One-Step® and its generic versions are available in drugstores and some supermarkets to anyone, without a prescription. However you should not use EC as your regular birth control because it does not work as well as regular birth control. EC is meant to be used only when your regular birth control does not work for some unexpected reason.

Which Types Of Birth Control Do I Have To See My Doctor To Get?

You need a prescription for these types of birth control:

- Oral contraceptives: the pill and the mini-pill (in some states, birth control pills are now available without a prescription, through the pharmacy)

- Patch

- Vaginal ring

- Diaphragms (your doctor or nurse needs to fit one to the shape of your vagina)

- Shot/injection (you get the shot at your doctor's office or family planning clinic)

- Cervical cap

- Implantable rod (inserted by a doctor in the office or clinic)

- IUD (inserted by a doctor in the office or clinic)

You will need surgery or a medical procedure for:

- Female sterilization (tubal ligation)

- Male sterilization (vasectomy)

- Tubal implant (Essure®)

How Can I Get Free Or Low-Cost Birth Control?

Under the Affordable Care Act (ACA) [the healthcare law], most insurance plans cover U.S. Food and Drug Administration (FDA)-approved prescription birth control for women, such as the pill, IUDs, and female sterilization, at no additional cost to you. This also includes birth control counseling.

- If you have insurance, check with your insurance provider to find out what is included in your plan.

- If you have Medicaid, your insurance covers birth control. This includes birth control prescriptions and visits to your doctor related to birth control. Programs vary between states, so check with your state's Medicaid program (www.medicaid.gov/medicaid/by-state/by-state.html) to learn what your benefits are.

- If you don't have insurance, don't panic. Family planning (reproductive health) clinics may provide some birth control methods for free or at low cost.

How Does Birth Control Work?

Birth control works to prevent pregnancy in different ways, depending upon the type of birth control you choose:

- **Female or male sterilization surgery** prevents the sperm from reaching the egg by cutting or damaging the tubes that carry sperm (in men) or eggs (in women).

- **Long-acting reversible contraceptives or "LARC" methods** (intrauterine devices, hormonal implants) prevent your ovaries from releasing eggs, prevent sperm from getting to the egg, or make implantation of the egg in the uterus (womb) unlikely.

- **Short-acting hormonal methods,** such as the pill, mini-pill, patch, shot, and vaginal ring, prevent your ovaries from releasing eggs or prevent sperm from getting to the egg.

- **Barrier methods,** such as condoms, diaphragms, sponge, cervical cap, prevent sperm from getting to the egg.

- **Natural rhythm methods** involve avoiding sex or using other forms of birth control on the days when you are most fertile (most likely to get pregnant).

Which Types Of Birth Control Help Prevent Sexually Transmitted Infections (STIs)?

Only two types can protect you from STIs, including human immunodeficiency virus (HIV): male condoms and female condoms.

While condoms are the best way to prevent STIs if you have sex, they are not the most effective type of birth control. If you have sex, the best way to prevent both STIs and pregnancy is to use what is called "dual protection." Dual protection means you use a condom to prevent STIs each time you have sex, and at the same time, you use a more effective form of birth control, such as an intrauterine device (IUD), implant, or shot.

In choosing a method of contraception, dual protection from the simultaneous risk for HIV and other sexually transmitted diseases (STDs) also should be considered. Although hormonal contraceptives and IUDs are highly effective at preventing pregnancy, they do not protect against STDs, including HIV. Consistent and correct use of the male latex condom reduces the risk for HIV infection and other STDs, including chlamydial infection, gonococcal infection, and trichomoniasis. Although evidence is limited, use of female condoms can provide protection from acquisition and transmission of STDs.

(Source: "U.S. Medical Eligibility Criteria For Contraceptive Use, 2016," Centers for Disease Control and Prevention (CDC).)

Are Birth Control Pills Safe?

Yes, hormonal birth control methods, such as the pill, are safe for most women. Today's birth control pills have lower doses of hormones than in the past. This has lowered the risk of side effects and serious health problems.

Today's birth control pills can have health benefits for some women, such as a lower risk of some kinds of cancer. Also, different brands and types of birth control pills (and other forms of hormonal birth control) can increase your risk for some health problems and side effects. Side effects can include weight gain, headaches, irregular bleeding, breast tenderness, and mood changes.

Talk to your doctor about whether hormonal birth control is right for you.

Does Birth Control Raise My Risk For Health Problems?

It can, depending on your health and the type of birth control you use. Talk to your doctor to find the birth control method that is right for you.

Different forms of birth control have different health risks and side effects. Some birth control methods that increase your risk for health problems include:

- **Hormonal birth control.** Combination birth control pills (birth control with both estrogen and progesterone) and some other forms of hormonal birth control, such as the vaginal ring or skin patch, may raise your risk for blood clots and high blood pressure. Blood clots and high blood pressure can cause a heart attack or stroke. A blood clot in the legs can also go to your lungs, causing serious damage or even death. These are serious side effects of hormonal birth control, but they are rare.

- **Spermicides (used alone or with the cervical cap, diaphragm or sponge).** Spermicides that have nonoxynol-9 can irritate the vagina. This can raise your risk for getting HIV. Use spermicides with nonoxynol-9 only if you are in a monogamous relationship (you have sex only with each other) with a man you know is HIV-negative. Also, medicines for vaginal yeast infections may make spermicides less effective.

- **IUDs.** IUDs can slightly raise your risk of an ectopic pregnancy. Ectopic pregnancies happen when a fertilized egg implants somewhere outside of the uterus (womb), usually in one of the fallopian tubes. An ectopic pregnancy is a serious medical problem that should be treated as soon as possible. IUDs also have a very rare but serious risk of infection or puncture of the uterus.

What Do I Do If I Miss A Day Taking The Pill?

Follow the instructions that came with your birth control about using back-up birth control (such as a condom and spermicide). You also can follow these recommendations from the Centers for Disease Control and Prevention (CDC).

If you are late or miss a day taking your pill:

- Take the late or missed pill as soon as possible.

- Continue taking the rest of your pills at your normal time, even if it means taking two pills on the same day.

- You do not need other forms of birth control, such as a condom, unless you need to protect against STIs.

If you miss two or more days in a row:

- Take only the most recent missed pill as soon as possible.

- Continue taking the rest of your pills at your normal time, even if it means taking two pills on the same day.

- Use back-up birth control, such as a condom and spermicide, or do not have sex until you have taken a pill for seven days in a row.

- If you missed pills during days in the last week of active pills (days 15–21 for 28-day pill packs), start a new pack the next day. If you are not able to start a new pack right away, use back-up birth control or avoid sex until hormone pills from a new pack have been taken for 7 days in a row.

- Consider emergency contraception if you missed pills during the first week and had sex.

Talk to your doctor if you continue to miss taking your birth control pill or find it hard to take the pill at the same time each day. You may want to consider a different type of birth control, such as an IUD, an implant, shot, ring, or patch that you don't have to remember to take every day.

How Effective Is The Withdrawal Method?

Not very! About 22 out of 100 women who use withdrawal as their only form of birth control for a year will get pregnant.

Withdrawal is when a man takes his penis out of a woman's vagina ("pulls out") before he ejaculates or "comes" (has an orgasm). This lowers the chance of sperm from going to the egg. "Pulling out" can be hard for a man to do. It takes a lot of self-control.

Even if you use withdrawal, sperm can be released before the man pulls out. When a man's penis first becomes erect, some fluid may be on the tip of the penis. This fluid has sperm in it, so you could still get pregnant. Withdrawal also does not protect you from STIs, including HIV.

Chapter 7
Teen Pregnancy And The Media

Teen pregnancy rates in the United States have dropped significantly since peaking in the early 1990s. In 2015 (the most recent year for which statistics are available), the rate was 22 births per 1,000 girls aged 15 to 19. That's a decline of 64 percent since the high point in 1991. Nevertheless, the United States teen pregnancy rate is the highest among developed nations, with more than 750,000 teenage pregnancies per year. And medical evidence shows that babies born to teens have a higher risk of health problems than those of older mothers. In addition, teen mothers are less likely to graduate from high school and attend college, while teen fathers also tend to be less educated and less likely to have a job than older parents.

Can Media Be A Negative Influence?

There's no question that we're all exposed to more media influences now than ever before. In addition to television, radio, and movies, the Internet and the explosion of social media have revolutionized the way we receive and process information. And many people believe that the portrayal of sex in popular media encourages teens to engage in sexual activity, which in turn may account for the high U.S. teenage pregnancy rate. Thus far, however, there hasn't been an abundance of research that conclusively links media influence to teen pregnancy.

One well-known study by the Rand Corporation found that frequent exposure to sexual content on television was associated with a significantly higher likelihood of teen pregnancy. For the study, researchers interviewed a nationwide sample of teens aged 12 to 17, concentrating on "23 popular programs that were widely available on broadcast and cable television and contained high levels of sexual content." (These included "Sex and the City" and "Friends.")

"Teen Pregnancy And The Media," © 2017 Omnigraphics. Reviewed March 2017.

The same teens were then interviewed again one year and again three years later. From the results, researchers estimated that teens who view high levels of televised sexual content are twice as likely to become pregnant or be responsible for a pregnancy than others of the same age group.

Since there hasn't been much other extensive research that's made a connection between sexual media content and teen pregnancy, a lot of sources have cited the Rand study as proof of this influence. However, the study's authors cautioned that other factors may also have had an effect on their findings, including the possibility that sexually active teens might seek out television shows with more sexual content. And a number of experts have cautioned against making this kind of connection between media content and the U.S. teen pregnancy rate.

Could Media Be A Positive Influence?

The other side of the coin is that certain media content might actually be a factor in reducing teen pregnancy. The National Campaign to Prevent Teen and Unplanned Pregnancy conducted a study that suggests exactly that. The nonprofit organization conducted a poll of young people aged 12 to 19, asking how they were influenced by television programs like "Teen Mom" and "Sixteen and Pregnant." The researchers found that 79 percent of girls and 67 percent of boys said the way characters on these shows deal with teen pregnancy made them "think more about their own risk of getting pregnant or causing a pregnancy and how to avoid it."

In addition, the study found that 76 percent of those interviewed said that media content depicting sex and relationship issues can be a good way to begin serious conversations with adults about those topics. And 93 percent said that through these shows they learned that pregnancy, childbirth, and dealing with a baby were harder than they had previously imagined.

Like the Rand study, this research also received a great deal of attention, with many sources citing it as evidence that media can, indeed, be a factor in reducing teen pregnancy. They believe that the more teens are exposed to the realities of dealing with pregnancy, childbirth, and childrearing at such a young age, the more they'll be inclined to be more thoughtful and careful about sexual activity. But, again, many experts note that concluding that these shows are directly responsible for the falling teen pregnancy rate is an oversimplification.

So, Can Media Influence Teen Pregnancy?

The simple answer is, there's no simple answer. Most experts agree that while the findings of these kinds of studies are interesting and provide useful information, no one has yet definitively proven a direct correlation between media and behavior—and that includes actions like speeding after watching a car chase or becoming violent after seeing an action movie, as well as a connection between media and sexual activity and pregnancy. And such a correlation is likely to be impossible to prove.

But one thing a large number of people do believe is that increased conversations about sex and pregnancy between teens and adults, and teens and their peers, can lead to heightened awareness of these issues and their potential consequences. And while sexual content in the media is often felt to be presented in a negative light—with depictions that include random casual sex, crude terminology, misogyny, and abusive relationships—some of this content can serve as a means of beginning conversations that can bring attention to these topics and perhaps those conversations can lead to positive behavior.

References

1. "Exposure to Sex on TV May Increase the Chance of Teen Pregnancy," Rand Corporation, 2008.

2. Grant, Christina, MD, FRCPC. "Teens, Sex and the Media: Is There a Connection?" *Paediatric Child Health*, May-June 2003.

3. "Is Media Glamorizing Teen Pregnancy?" PRnewswire.com, October 4, 2010.

4. Kalenga, Erick. "The Influence Television Has on Teen Pregnancy," Dailyprogress.com, February 2, 2014.

5. "Media," National Campaign to Prevent Teen and Unplanned Pregnancy, n.d.

6. Nauert, Rick, PhD. "TV Sex Influences Teen Pregnancy," Psychcentral.com, October 6, 2015.

7. Silvers, Hillary. "Does Media Affect Teen Pregnancy?" More.com, 2016.

Part Two
If You Think You're Pregnant

Chapter 8

Finding Out If You're Pregnant

Common Signs Of Pregnancy

The primary sign of pregnancy is missing a menstrual period or two or more consecutive periods, but many women experience other symptoms of pregnancy before they notice a missed period.

Missing a period does not always mean a woman is pregnant. Menstrual irregularities are common and can have a variety of causes, including taking birth control pills, conditions such as diabetes and polycystic ovary syndrome, eating disorders, excessive exercise, and certain medications. Women who miss a period should see their healthcare provider to find out whether they are pregnant or whether they have a specific health problem.

Pregnancy symptoms vary from woman to woman. A woman may experience every common symptom, just a few, or none at all. Some signs of early pregnancy include:

- **Slight bleeding.** One study shows as many as 25 percent of pregnant women experience slight bleeding or spotting that is lighter in color than normal menstrual blood. This typically occurs at the time of implantation of the fertilized egg (about 6 to 12 days after conception) but is common in the first 12 weeks of pregnancy.

- **Tender, swollen breasts or nipples.** Women may notice this symptom as early as 1 to 2 weeks after conception. Hormonal changes can make the breasts sore or even tingly. The breasts feel fuller or heavier as well.

About This Chapter: Text under the heading "Common Signs Of Pregnancy" is excerpted from "What Are Some Common Signs Of Pregnancy?" *Eunice Kennedy Shriver* National Institute of Child Health and Human Development (NICHD), December 5, 2012. Reviewed March 2017; Text under the heading "Home Pregnancy Tests" is excerpted from "Pregnancy," U.S. Food and Drug Administration (FDA), June 5, 2014.

- **Fatigue.** Many women feel more tired early in pregnancy because their bodies are producing more of a hormone called progesterone, which helps maintain the pregnancy and encourages the growth of milk-producing glands in the breasts. In addition, during pregnancy the body pumps more blood to carry nutrients to the fetus. Pregnant women may notice fatigue as early as 1 week after conception.

- **Headaches.** The sudden rise of hormones may trigger headaches early in pregnancy.

- **Nausea or vomiting.** This symptom can start anywhere from 2 to 8 weeks after conception and can continue throughout pregnancy. Commonly referred to as "morning sickness," it can actually occur at any time during the day.

- **Food cravings or aversions.** Sudden cravings or developing a dislike of favorite foods are both common throughout pregnancy. A food craving or aversion can last the entire pregnancy or vary throughout this period.

- **Mood swings.** Hormonal changes during pregnancy often cause sharp mood swings. These can occur as early as a few weeks after conception.

- **Frequent urination.** The need to empty the bladder more often is common throughout pregnancy. In the first few weeks of pregnancy, the body produces a hormone called human chorionic gonadotropin, which increases blood flow to the pelvic region, causing women to have to urinate more often.

Many of these symptoms can also be a sign of another condition, the result of changing birth control pills, or stress, and thus they do not always mean that a woman is pregnant. Women should see their healthcare provider if they suspect they are pregnant.

A missed period is often the first clue that a woman might be pregnant. Sometimes, a woman might suspect she is pregnant even sooner. Symptoms such as headache, fatigue, and breast tenderness, can occur even before a missed period. The wait to know can be emotional. These days, many women first use home pregnancy tests (HPT) to find out. Your doctor also can test you.

(Source: "Knowing If You Are Pregnant," Office on Women's Health (OWH), U.S. Department of Health and Human Services (HHS).)

Home Pregnancy Tests
What Does This Test Do?

This is a home-use test kit to measure human chorionic gonadotropin (hCG) in your urine. You produce this hormone only when you are pregnant.

What Is hCG?

hCG is a hormone produced by your placenta when you are pregnant. It appears shortly after the embryo attaches to the wall of the uterus. If you are pregnant, this hormone increases very rapidly. If you have a 28 day menstrual cycle, you can detect hCG in your urine 12–15 days after ovulation.

What Type Of Test Is This?

This is a qualitative test—you find out whether or not you have elevated hCG levels indicating that you are pregnant.

Why Should You Do This Test?

You should use this test to find out if you are pregnant.

How Accurate Is This Test?

The accuracy of this test depends on how well you follow the instructions and interpret the results. If you mishandle or misunderstand the test kit, you may get poor results.

Most pregnancy tests have about the same ability to detect hCG, but their ability to show whether or not you are pregnant depends on how much hCG you are producing. If you test too early in your cycle or too close to the time you became pregnant, your placenta may **not** have had enough time to produce hCG. This would mean that you are pregnant but you got a **negative** test result.

Because many women have irregular periods, and women may miscalculate when their period is due, 10 to 20 pregnant women out of every 100 will not detect their pregnancy on the first day of their missed period.

How Do You Do This Test?

For most home pregnancy tests (HPT), you either hold a test strip in your urine stream or you collect your urine in a cup and dip your test strip into the cup. If you are pregnant, most test strips produce a colored line, but this will depend on the brand you purchased. Read the instructions for the test you bought and follow them carefully. Make sure you know how to get good results. The test usually takes only about 5 minutes.

The different tests for sale vary in their abilities to detect low levels of hCG. For the most reliable results, test 1–2 weeks after you miss your period. There are some tests for sale that are sensitive enough to show you are pregnant before you miss your period.

You can improve your chances for an accurate result by using your first morning urine for the test. If you are pregnant, it will have more hCG in it than later urines. If you think you are pregnant, but your first test was negative, you can take the test again after several days. Since the amount of hCG increases rapidly when you are pregnant, you may get a positive test on later days. Some test kits come with more than one test in them to allow you to repeat the test.

Is This Test Similar To The One My Doctor Uses?

The home pregnancy test and the test your doctor uses are similar in their abilities to detect hCG, however your doctor is probably more experienced in running the test. If you produce only a small amount of hCG, your doctor may not be able to detect it any better than you could. Your doctor may also use a blood test to see if you are pregnant. Finally, your doctor may have more information about you from your history, physical exam, and other tests that may give a more reliable result.

Does A Positive Test Mean You Are Pregnant?

Usually, yes, but you must be sure to read and interpret the results correctly.

Some medicines affect HPTs. Discuss the medicines you use with your doctor before trying to become pregnant.

(Source: "Knowing If You Are Pregnant," Office on Women's Health (OWH), U.S. Department of Health and Human Services (HHS).)

Do Negative Test Results Mean That You Are Not Pregnant?

No, there are several reasons why you could receive false negative test results. If you tested too early in your cycle, your placenta may not have had time to produce enough hCG for the test to detect. Or, you may not have waited long enough before you took this test.

If you have a negative result, you would be wise to consider this a tentative finding. You should not use medications and should consider avoiding potentially harmful behaviors, such as smoking or drinking alcohol, until you have greater certainty that you are not pregnant.

You will probably recognize incorrect results with the passage of time. You may detect false negatives by the unexpected onset of menses (regular vaginal bleeding associated with "periods"). Repeat testing and/or other investigations such as ultrasound may provide corrected results.

Chapter 9
Telling Parents You're Pregnant

If you've just learned you're pregnant, you're not alone.

You might feel confused, scared, or shocked by the news. You might think, "This can't really be happening." You promise yourself you'll be so much more careful in the future. And you know you'll probably have to tell your parents.

Preparing To Talk To Parents

No matter how close you are to your parents, you're going to wonder how they'll react. It's one thing if your parents realize you're having sex and they're OK with that. But it's another thing if they've forbidden you to date or if having premarital sex is completely against their values and beliefs.

Everyone's Situation Is Different
Lots of things will influence how a parent reacts to news of your pregnancy, such as:

- how surprised or shocked your parents might be to learn you've been having sex
- your parents' values about dating, sex, and pregnancy
- your parents' expectations or rules for you
- your parents' feelings about your partner and your relationship
- your age or maturity level

About This Chapter: Text in this chapter is © 1995–2017. The Nemours Foundation/KidsHealth®. Reprinted with permission.

Most parents fall somewhere in the middle. For example, some parents have pretty liberal values but they're still shocked to learn their teen had sex. Even parents who know their teens are having sex can still be disappointed or worried about their future.

Your parents' personalities also play a part in how they'll react. Some parents are easy to talk to or calmer in a crisis. Some are more emotional, more easily stressed out, more likely to get upset or angry, to yell or cry, or express themselves loudly.

Most parents want to be supportive of a daughter who is pregnant (or a son who got a girl pregnant), even if they are angry or upset at first. But a few may react violently to the news and let anger get out of control.

Some parents don't show how they feel at first. They may take time to absorb the news. Others react quickly and there's no mistaking how they feel. Some will listen and be sensitive to your feelings. Some parents will spring into action, taking charge and telling you what to do.

Think about how your parents have reacted to other situations. Try to imagine how they might respond—but remember it's impossible to really know for sure. Still, thinking about what to expect can help you feel prepared for the conversation you plan to have.

The Conversation

First, find the words. You might say, "I have something difficult to tell you. I found out that I'm pregnant." Then wait. Allow your parents to absorb what you said.

Be prepared to deal with the reaction. What happens next? Will your parents be angry, stressed, or emotional? Will they lecture you? Use harsh words? Ask a ton of questions?

It's good to think ahead about what you might do and how you may feel. For instance, if a parent yells, you'll want to be prepared so you can keep the conversation productive and resist any urge to yell back.

Of course, not every parent yells. Many don't. Even if parents have a strong reaction at first, most want to help their children. Lots of teens are surprised at how supportive their parents turn out to be.

It can help to tell your parents that you understand their feelings and point of view. Saying things like, "I know you're really mad," "I know this isn't what you wanted for me," or, "I know this isn't what you expected" can help your parents be more understanding. The key is to be honest and speak from the heart. If you say what you think parents want to hear or make statements just to calm them, it might sound fake.

Give your parents time to speak without jumping in. Listen to what they say. Let them vent if they have to.

Tell them how you feel. Part of your conversation might involve telling parents how you feel. For example, if you know you've disappointed them and you feel sorry about it, say that. Let them know if you feel disappointed in yourself, too.

You might say, "Mom and Dad, I know I've disappointed you. I know you're upset. I'm really sorry for putting you through this. I'm disappointed in myself, too."

Share your fears and worries, such as, "I'm scared about how I'm going to handle this, what my friends will think, and what it means about school." Or, "I can't believe this is happening to me and I'm not sure what to do."

Putting your feelings into words takes plenty of maturity and it's not easy to do. Don't worry if the words don't come out perfectly or if you cry or get emotional as you're saying them. It can help to think about your feelings ahead of time. If you can't imagine expressing your feelings out loud, consider writing them down in a letter.

If you need to, get help breaking the news. A visit to your doctor's office or a health clinic is a must—not just for your health, but to get more information and discuss the realities of your situation. You'll want to understand your choices and explore your feelings with an experienced professional. During your visit, the doctor, nurse, or health counselor also can help you think through how to tell your parents. If you want, they could even be there as you talk to your parents.

Talking About Your Decisions

Now that you've told your parents, you'll have some important decisions to make. Talking decisions over with others can help. Sometimes parents—including your boyfriend's parents—can offer a new angle or ideas.

Whatever you decide, it needs to be what you want, not what someone else wants you to do. That's especially true if you think most of the child-raising will fall to you. It's a big job.

Becoming a teen parent affects your education, job, and financial future—and often your boyfriend's too. Over half of teen pregnancies end with the birth of the baby. Some teens decide to keep the baby. Others let someone adopt the child. Some teen pregnancies end in miscarriage, and about one third end in abortion.

Talking about your options isn't easy, especially if none of them is what you had in mind. Some families need the help of a counselor to talk about this difficult and complicated situation in a way that lets everyone be respected and heard.

It's More Than Just Breaking the News

Talking to a parent about your pregnancy takes more than just one conversation. In the coming months, you'll probably have many different feelings all at once. Sometimes, you might feel shock and disbelief. Other times, you may be scared or worried. You may feel sad, guilty, or angry at yourself. At times, you might also feel excited and happy.

Some days you might be ready for what's ahead. Other days, you may feel totally unprepared and confused. You'll have many emotions to sort through and it will take time. It helps if you can talk to a parent about all these thoughts and feelings.

Protecting Yourself

To some parents, the news that you're having a baby will feel like a terrible crisis. Depending on their beliefs, cultural values, or personalities, parents might feel shame, guilt, or embarrassment. They might feel angry and assign blame. Sometimes parents scream, yell, and use putdowns. In some cases, anger can get out of control.

You know your parent and you know your situation. If you need to tell your parents you're pregnant but think they might react in a way that could hurt you, have someone else with you when you tell them. If you're concerned about your safety, get advice. A teen health clinic, such as Planned Parenthood, or a teen pregnancy hotline can guide you and steer you toward resources to support you.

Of course, most parents won't react with extreme anger. The thing to remember is every parent is different and you know yours best.

When Parents Have Your Back

Talking to parents whenever you can is a good way to sort through the many feelings and issues that arise. In the best of situations, parents can help you make important decisions and support your choices. They can be a source of guidance and encouragement.

Sometimes a difficult situation brings people closer and strengthens their bonds. Sometimes, however unexpectedly, a difficult situation can help a family discover unconditional love, support, kindness, forgiveness, acceptance, teamwork, and optimism.

Chapter 10
Thinking About Abortion

There are two kinds of abortion in the U.S.—in-clinic abortion and the abortion pill.

Abortions are very common. In fact, 3 out of 10 women in the U.S. have an abortion by the time they are 45 years old.

If you are pregnant, you have options. If you are trying to decide if abortion is the right choice for you, you probably have many things to think about. Learning the facts about abortion may help you in making your decision.

If you are under 18, your state may require one or both of your parents to give permission for your abortion or be told of your decision prior to the abortion. However, in most states you can ask a judge to excuse you from these requirements.

Only you can decide what is best for you. But we are here to help. A staff member at your local Planned Parenthood health center can discuss abortion and all of your options with you and help you find the services you need.

The Abortion Pill At A Glance

- Take medicines to end an early pregnancy

- Safe and effective

- Available from many Planned Parenthood health centers

- Costs up to $800, but often less

About This Chapter: Text in this chapter is excerpted from "Abortion," © 2017 Planned Parenthood Federation of America Inc. Reprinted with permission.

A woman has many decisions to make when considering abortion. If you're thinking about abortion, your health care provider may talk with you about a few different abortion methods. You may be offered the option to have an in-clinic abortion procedure. Or you may be offered the option to have a medication abortion by taking the abortion pill. Medication abortion is the kind of abortion discussed on this chapter.

Whether you're thinking about having a medication abortion, you're concerned about a woman who may be having one, or you're someone who's just curious about medication abortion, you may have many questions. Here are some of the most common questions we hear women ask about the abortion pill. We hope you find the answers helpful. And if you're thinking of having a medication abortion, we hope they help you decide what is best for you.

If you are under 18, your state may require one or both of your parents to give permission for your abortion or be told of your decision prior to the abortion. However, in most states you can ask a judge to excuse you from these requirements. Learn more about parental consent for abortion.

What Is The Abortion Pill?

Medication abortion—also called the abortion pill—is a safe and effective way to end an early pregnancy.

How Does The Abortion Pill Work?

"Abortion pill" is the popular name for using two different medicines to end a pregnancy: mifepristone and misoprostol.

Your doctor or nurse will give you the first pill, mifepristone, at the clinic. Pregnancy needs a hormone called progesterone to grow normally. Mifepristone blocks your body's own progesterone. You'll also get some antibiotics.

You take the second medicine, misoprostol, 24-48 hours later, usually at home. This medicine causes cramping and bleeding to empty the uterus. It's kind of like having a really heavy, crampy period, and the process is very similar to an early miscarriage.

How Effective Is The Abortion Pill?

The abortion pill is very effective. For people who are 8 weeks pregnant or less, it works about 98 out of 100 times. From 8-9 weeks pregnant, it works about 96 out of 100 times. From 9-10 weeks, it works 93 out of 100 times.

The abortion pill usually works, but if it doesn't, you can take more medicine or have an in-clinic abortion to complete the abortion.

When Can I Take The Abortion Pill?

You usually can get a medication abortion up to 70 days (10 weeks) after the first day of your last period. If it has been 71 days or more since the first day of your last period, you can have an in-clinic abortion to end your pregnancy.

Why Do People Choose The Abortion Pill?

Which kind of abortion you choose all depends on your personal preference and situation. With medication abortion, some people like that you don't need to have a procedure in a doctor's office. You can have your medication abortion at home or in another comfortable place that you choose. You get to decide who you want to be with during your abortion, or you can go it alone. Because medication abortion is similar to a miscarriage, many people feel like it's more "natural" and less invasive.

Your doctor, nurse, or health center staff can help you decide which kind of abortion is best for you.

In-Clinic Abortion Procedures At A Glance

- Medical procedures that end pregnancy
- Safe and effective
- Available from many Planned Parenthood health centers
- Costs up to $1,500 in the first trimester, but often less

A woman has many decisions to make when considering abortion. If you're thinking about abortion, your health care provider may talk with you about a few different abortion methods. You may be offered the option to have an in-clinic abortion procedure, which is the kind of abortion discussed on this page. Or you may be offered the abortion pill.

Whether you're thinking about having an in-clinic abortion, you're concerned about a woman who may be having one, or you're someone who's just curious about abortion methods, you may have many questions. Here are some of the most common questions we hear women ask about in-clinic abortions. We hope you find the answers helpful. And if you're thinking of having an in-clinic abortion procedure, we hope they help you decide what is best for you.

If you are under 18, your state may require one or both of your parents to give permission for your abortion or be told of your decision prior to the abortion. However, in most states you can ask a judge to excuse you from these requirements.

What Is An Abortion?

Abortion is a medical procedure that ends a pregnancy. In-clinic abortion procedures are safe and effective. In-clinic abortions are also called surgical abortions.

What Are The Types Of In-Clinic Abortions?

In-clinic abortion works by using suction to take a pregnancy out of your uterus. There are a couple of kinds of in-clinic abortion procedures. Your doctor or nurse will know which type is right for you, depending on how far you are into your pregnancy.

Suction abortion (also called vacuum aspiration) is the most common type of in-clinic abortion. It uses gentle suction to empty your uterus. It's usually used until about 14-16 weeks after your last period.

Dilation and Evacuation (D&E) is another kind of in-clinic abortion procedure. It uses suction and medical tools to empty your uterus. You can get a D&E later in a pregnancy than aspiration abortion—usually if it has been 16 weeks or longer since your last period.

How Effective Are In-Clinic Abortions?

In-clinic abortions are extremely effective. They work more than 99 out of every 100 times. Needing to get a repeat procedure because the abortion didn't work is really rare.

When Can I Get An In-Clinic Abortion?

How early you can get an abortion depends on where you go. In some places, you can get it as soon as you have a positive pregnancy test. Other doctors or nurses prefer to wait until 5-6 weeks after the first day of your last period.

How late you can get an abortion depends on the laws in your state and what doctor, abortion clinic, or Planned Parenthood health center you go to. It may be harder to find a health care provider who will do an abortion after the 12th week of pregnancy, so it's best to try to have your abortion as soon as possible.

Why Do People Choose An In-Clinic Abortion?

Which kind of abortion you choose all depends on your personal preference and situation. Some people choose in-clinic abortion because they want to have their procedure done at a health center, with nurses, doctors, and trained support staff there the whole time. (With the abortion pill, you have the abortion at home.)

In-clinic abortions are also much faster than the abortion pill: most in-clinic abortions only take about 5-10 minutes, while a medication abortion may take up to 24 hours to complete.

Your nurse, doctor, or health center counselor can help you decide which kind of abortion is best for you.

Parental Consent And Notification Laws

If you're under 18, you may or may not have to tell a parent in order to get an abortion—it all depends on the laws where you live.

Some states don't have any laws about telling your parents or getting their permission. But some states say you have to get permission from a parent or older family member to have an abortion. Other states don't make you get permission, but your parents will have to know that you're getting an abortion.

A judge may be able to excuse you from having to tell your parents or get their permission—this is called "judicial bypass."

The exact rules are different in different places. Find information on parental involvement in your state below.

And know that you're not alone. If you're pregnant and want to have an abortion, call your nearest Planned Parenthood health center as soon as possible. They can help explain the laws in your state, let you know what your options are, and give you tips on talking with your parents.

It's important to take action right away. Abortion is very safe, but there are more risks the longer you wait. There are also time limits on abortion in some states. And if you need a judicial bypass, it can take a while to get through the process.

Chapter 11
Thinking About Adoption

Adoption is a process—with legal, social, and emotional aspects—in which children who will not be raised by their birth parents become permanent legal members of another family. When it comes to adoption, there is no one right decision for everyone. Understanding adoption—including why others choose adoption or not and its long-term impact—may help you figure out what's right for you and your child.

Why Do Some Expectant Parents Choose To Place Their Baby For Adoption?

Everyone's situation is different, but many women (and their partners) choose adoption because they do not feel ready or able to raise a child. They often believe that the baby will have a better life in an adoptive home with parents who are ready to welcome and care for a child. As such, these mothers typically feel that they are putting their baby's best interests ahead of their own. Other factors that sometimes play a part in parents' decisions to place their children for adoption include money problems, personal goals, and family attitudes.

Why Do Some Expectant Parents Choose To Raise Their Baby Rather Than Place The Baby For Adoption?

Women experiencing an unplanned pregnancy (and their partners) who consider adoption but decide to raise their child themselves may do so because they conclude that they have the commitment and support necessary to raise a child. They may feel that maintaining their connection with their child and preventing a profound loss for themselves and their child

About This Chapter: This chapter includes text excerpted from "Are You Pregnant And Thinking About Adoption?" Child Welfare Information Gateway, U.S. Department of Health and Human Services (HHS), February 2014.

outweigh any possible advantages of adoption. Some birth parents who were unsure before their child's birth find they do feel ready to be a parent after they've held and connected with their baby.

What Is The Impact Of The Adoption Decision?

Adoption is more than a one-time legal event; adoption is a lifelong process with long-term impact for everyone involved (your child, you and your family members, the birth father and his relatives, and the adoptive family). Once an adoption is legally finalized, it is permanent, and it will change your relationship with your child forever. In the eyes of the law, your child is no longer related to you. The adoptive parents will raise your child and have full legal rights and responsibilities as the child's parents. While experiences differ, many birth parents who place their child for adoption experience feelings of loss, grief, and guilt. For some, it is a traumatic experience. These feelings may persist many years after the adoption and may negatively affect birth parents' later lives and relationships.

Keep In Mind
While birth parents and children who have been adopted often struggle with identity issues and lifelong feelings of loss and grief, many will learn how to work through these emotions, often with the help of counseling.

If I Choose Adoption, Will I Know What Happens To My Child?

Placing a child for adoption does not mean necessarily that you won't have any future contact with your child. In past generations, many adoptions were surrounded in secrecy, and communication between birth parents and their children was discouraged. Today, most infant adoptions have some degree of openness in which birth parents have some contact with adoptive parents and their children who have been adopted.

When Do I Have To Make My Decision?

Most State laws require that the final decision to place a child for adoption be made after the baby is born. Think of it as making the adoption decision twice—once while you are pregnant and again after giving birth. After consideration of your options, you may prepare for adoption by selecting a licensed adoption agency or adoption lawyer and selecting adoptive parents (or parent). Nevertheless, the final and legal decision is made by you (or you and the father) after the child's birth.

Do Remember

It's hard to know exactly how you'll feel after the birth of your baby. **You should not sign papers that make the adoption final until you are sure of your decision.** Until the final papers are signed, you have parental rights to make decisions regarding your child.

Gathering Information And Exploring Your Options

Gathering information, consulting with others, and thoughtfully exploring all your options will help you make a fully informed decision. Reading this chapter can get you started. Other sources of information and support are described below.

- **The Internet.** If you are just beginning to research your options, the Internet can be helpful. You can explore the Internet using search terms such as "unplanned pregnancy," "adoption options," "parenting," and "adoption birth mother" (or "birth father") to name a few. Try to visit trustworthy websites. You also may want to look at blogs and discussion forums that include first-person accounts and may provide insights into the adoption process and what others have experienced.

Information on the web can be biased or inaccurate. Try to look at several websites and blogs and note varied points of view as well as common themes. In addition, be aware that some dishonest online groups may try to take advantage of pregnant women at a vulnerable time.

- **Books.** Like the Internet, books can let you find and digest information in private. To get a complete view of adoption, you may want to look at books that present different perspectives, including those of parents who placed their children for adoption, parents who adopted children, children and adults who were adopted, and parents raising children in specific situations (for example, single parents or teen parents).

- **Trusted friends and family members.** It can be helpful to talk through your feelings and options with a trusted family member or friend. Try to find someone who will listen and won't pressure you into making a decision that doesn't feel right.

While it's good to talk things through with friends and family, ultimately, the decision is yours to make.

- **Counselors.** A trained counselor can help you to not only understand your options and their long-term implications, but also explore your feelings about those options. You can find professional counselors—including therapists and social workers—at public departments of social services, local health or mental health centers and hospitals, and adoption agencies. Counselors also may be religious leaders, including pastors, rabbis, or others associated with a place of worship. Your doctor, friends, or family members may be able to refer you to a professional counselor. Referral services also can be found through local United Way organizations. (Try calling 211 or visiting www.211us.org.) No matter where you go, look for a counselor who is experienced in working with pregnant women and who treats you with sensitivity and respect.

> It's important to find a counselor who can answer your questions in an unbiased way and who doesn't stand to gain from the decision you make. Some counselors may be predisposed toward one option (for example, due to professional affiliations), or they may have other people's interests in mind (for example, prospective adoptive parents waiting to find an infant available for adoption). As such, some women prefer to find counselors that are not associated with an adoption agency or lawyer to lessen the likelihood of being pressured toward adoption.

- **Adoption agencies and adoption lawyers.** If you are leaning toward adoption, talking with someone at a licensed adoption agency or with a lawyer who specializes in adoption may be helpful to learn more about the adoption process.

> Talking to an agency or lawyer does not mean that you're promising to place your child for adoption but rather serves as another way to collect information. Do not sign any legal papers until you have made up your mind to develop an adoption plan.

Making The Adoption Decision: Questions To Ask Yourself

The decision to place a child for adoption is never easy. Like the decision to parent a child, it takes courage and love. Following are some questions that you may want to think about as you make your decision.

Have I Explored All My Options?

While you may be leaning in one direction, it's important that you take time and explore all of your options. The options that "rise to the top" may vary depending on your circumstances and beliefs. Carefully assess the benefits and challenges of each option, as well as potential supports to address any challenges. Are you thinking about adoption only because you have current money problems or because your living situation is difficult? If so, there may be other answers. Have you asked friends and family if they can help? Have you looked into local programs or called Social Services to see what they can do? Social workers may be able to help you find a way to parent your baby by assisting with finding a place to live, child care, job training, or other supports. Alternatively, have you considered placing your child (formally or informally) with a family member? If you want more time to make your decision, have you asked an adoption agency whether there are any short-term options available (for example, temporary foster care)?

Have I Involved The Baby's Father In The Decision-Making Process?

There are several reasons for involving the baby's father, not the least of which are fathers' rights and State laws about fathers' roles and responsibilities in adoption. Most States require that the father (or the man you think is the father) be told about the baby before the adoption. This is true even if you aren't married to the father. While laws vary, your State's law may require that your baby's father (or your husband) sign legal papers agreeing to the adoption—granting legal "consent"—before you can place your child for adoption. In some cases where agencies and lawyers have pushed through adoptions without getting the father's consent, the court has legally overturned the adoption. Note also that, in some States, if parents are unmarried, the presumed father (or "putative" father) has a certain amount of time to put his name on the State's putative father registry or take other legal action to claim that he is the baby's father. If you don't know the father's name or whereabouts, some States require that a notice be published.

> Laws related to the father's role and responsibilities in adoption differ from State to State. To learn more about the laws in your State, visit www.childwelfare.gov/adoption/birth/for/legal.cfm or ask an adoption lawyer or an adoption agency staff member to explain the legal requirements to you.

If you have a good relationship with your baby's father, you may be able to help each other with considering the options and making a decision. Some women considering adoption, however, do not have a good relationship with their child's father. For example, they may have had a violent relationship with the father. In such circumstances, you can ask an adoption agency or attorney to contact the father rather than deal with him directly.

67

Regardless of your relationship with your child's father, it's also important to think about your child's future perspective. At some point, most children who have been adopted ask questions about their birth parents and the circumstances of their adoption. Many will want to develop a relationship with their birth father. An adopted person who finds out that his or her birth mother made the adoption decision without consulting the birth father may feel tremendous resentment toward the birth mother.

Have I Talked About This Decision With My Own Family And The Father's Family?

Your family and/or the father's family may be a source of support as you consider what to do, even if the pregnancy has put a strain on your relationships. Besides emotional support, your families may be able to provide money, housing, and other kinds of help. In addition, if you are under 18 years of age, in some States your own parent(s) may also have to give permission for you to place your baby for adoption.

If you decide to go ahead with adoption, there may be someone in your family or the father's family who would like to adopt your baby. Kinship adoption can help maintain the child's connections to his or her family members and cultural heritage.

How Might I Feel In 10 Or 20 Years If I Place My Child For Adoption Or I Parent My Child Myself?

While it's impossible to know for sure how you will feel many years from now, you should consider the long-term effects of any decision you make. For instance, you may want to think about your future with and without this child. How would raising a child or placing a child for adoption affect what you want from life? What support systems may be needed to achieve your long-term plans under each of your options? How might you feel if you go on to have other children, or if you do not have any additional children?

There are no "right" or "wrong" responses to these questions, and you may not know the answers right now.

Chapter 12

Thinking About Parenting

Millions of women face unplanned pregnancies every year. If you are deciding what to do about an unplanned pregnancy, you have a lot to think about. You have three options—abortion, adoption, and parenting.

Whether you're thinking about parenting, you're helping a woman decide if parenting is right for her, or you're just curious about parenting, you may have many questions. Here are some of the most common questions we hear women ask when considering becoming a parent. We hope you find the answers helpful.

How Can I Know If Parenting Is The Right Option For Me?

We all have many important decisions to make in life. What to do about an unplanned pregnancy is an important and common decision faced by women. In fact, about half of all women in the U.S. have an unplanned pregnancy at some point in their lives. About 6 out of 10 women with unplanned pregnancies decide to continue their pregnancies.

Every woman's situation is different, and only you can decide what is best in your case. If you're trying to decide if parenting is the right option for you, you may find it helpful to list the advantages and disadvantages of having a child. Think about what advantages or disadvantages are most important to you. Consider your feelings and values about raising a child, and what you want for your life and for your family or future family.

About This Chapter: Text in this chapter is excerpted from "Thinking About Parenting," © 2017 Planned Parenthood Federation of America Inc. Reprinted with permission.

Some Things To Ask Yourself If You Are Thinking About Raising A Child

- Am I ready to help a child feel wanted and loved?
- Am I ready to cope with a tighter budget, less time for myself, and more stress?
- Do I have the support of family and friends?
- Am I ready to accept responsibility for all my child's needs?
- Would I prefer to have a child at another time?
- Is anyone pressuring me to continue or end the pregnancy?
- How do I feel about other women who have children from unplanned pregnancies?
- Can I afford to have a child?
- What would it mean for my future and my family's future if I had a child now?
- How important is it to me what other people will think about my decision?
- Can I handle the experience of pregnancy and raising a child?

If you are already a parent, ask yourself how bringing another child into your family will affect your other children. Think about what your answers mean to you. You may want to discuss your answers with your partner, someone in your family, a friend, a trusted religious adviser, or a counselor.

What Are Some Of The Advantages And Disadvantages Of Parenting?

Though parenting is hard work, it brings many rewards. Being a parent can be exciting and deeply rewarding. It can help you grow, understand yourself better, and enhance your life. Parents can feel delight at their child's accomplishments and the love and bond they share. Many people say that parenting brings great happiness and a deeper understanding of themselves.

But parents often give up a lot for their children. Meeting a child's needs can be very challenging. Parents deal with less sleep and less time to do the things they need and want to do. Having a baby is expensive, and many people find it hard to support their children. Having children can also put a parent's school plans or career on hold.

Many people find that having a child can test even the strongest relationship. And if you are single parenting, you may find it more difficult to find and keep a relationship.

If you already have children, you know firsthand both the joys and challenges parenting can bring. A child will change your life, whether it is your first child or not. If you don't have any children, talking with other parents about their daily lives with their children may help give you an idea about what you could expect.

Who Can Help Me Decide?

Most women look to their husbands, partners, families, health care providers, clergy, or someone else they trust for support as they make their decision about an unplanned pregnancy. Even though the decision about what to do about your pregnancy is up to you, most women find they'd also like to talk with trusted people in their lives to help them make up their minds.

If you need help deciding, specially trained educators at women's health clinics—like your Planned Parenthood health center—can talk it through with you. They can talk with you in private or you may bring someone with you if you wish. When looking for someone to talk with about your options, beware of so-called "crisis pregnancy centers." They are run by people who are against abortion, and who will not give you information about all of your options.

How Soon Do I Have to Decide?

Whether you choose adoption or to become a parent, if there is a chance that you will continue the pregnancy, you should begin prenatal care as soon as possible. You should have a medical exam early in your pregnancy—and regularly throughout your pregnancy—to make sure that you are healthy and the pregnancy is normal.

Even though most women have safe and healthy pregnancies, there are certain risks of pregnancy for a woman. They range from discomforts, such as nausea, fatigue, and aches and pains, to more serious risks, such as blood clots, high blood pressure, and diabetes. In extremely rare cases, complications can be fatal. That's why early and regular prenatal care is very important.

It may be important to take your time and think carefully about your decision. But you may not want to wait too long. If you are considering abortion, you should know that abortion is very safe, but the risks increase the longer a pregnancy goes on.

Can I Meet A Child's Needs?

Children have many needs. Your child will depend on you—for food, shelter, safety, affection, and guidance.

Parenting requires lots of love, energy, and patience. It is often complicated and frustrating. Your child's needs will constantly change and so will your ability to meet those needs. There will be times when you may feel that you are not doing a good job at parenting. To feel good about being a parent, it must be what you want to do—for a long time.

If you are thinking about becoming a parent, you may wonder if you are prepared. Do you have what you might need to take care of a child?

- Time—children can put your school plans or career on hold.

- Energy and care—children need parents who are loving, patient, and flexible.

- Planning—having children takes daily planning, as well as long-term planning for the next stages of the child's life.

- Material things and money—children need clothes, diapers, food, and health care, and they often need day care.

What Support Will I Need If I Have A Child?

Parenting is hard work—whether you are single and parenting or parenting with a partner, and whether it is your first child or another child in the family. A child requires nonstop care, and having a partner or other family member to share the work of parenting can make the job much easier.

New parents, whether they are single or in a couple, need support from lots of places. Worries about money and time are common for parents, and every family needs support now and then. Sometimes that might be grocery shopping, hand-me-down clothes, babysitting time, or just someone to talk with.

Single Parenting

Many people find themselves single parenting, or choose to become single parents. Single parenting can be very challenging, but it's certainly not impossible.

If you're thinking of single parenting, talk with family and friends about the help you will need. Find out how much time, energy, and money the people in your life are willing to give to you and your baby. If you will need money, be realistic about how much your friends and family can give. Some people will be able to help a lot, while others will be only able to help a little. If you need government support, keep in mind that it will only cover part of what you will need.

But being a single parent has its advantages, too. Because you will not have to make compromises with a partner, you can raise the child as you wish—with your values, principles, and beliefs.

Parenting With A Partner

A partnership can provide parents with much-needed support. Many couples find great satisfaction in sharing the responsibility of raising a child. They find their love and commitment to each other is made deeper by their shared love for their child.

However, parenting can also put stress on relationships. Parents may disagree about what is best for a child. If you have a baby, your relationship with your partner will change. Joint parenting takes good communication and a solid commitment in hard times.

When Extra Support Is Needed

Women often have a wide range of emotions after giving birth. The joy of a new baby can be mixed with feelings of sadness and anxiety, and feelings of being overwhelmed. Childbirth causes sudden shifts in hormones that can cause these feelings. You may need some extra support if you suffer from the "baby blues" during your baby's first few days or weeks.

Long-term depression is more common if a woman has a history of emotional problems or if she does not have supportive people in her life. Women should seek help from a health care provider or counselor if depression lasts more than two weeks or keeps them from doing what they need to do each day.

Overall, having lots of support from other people will be a big help to you if you decide to become a parent. Thinking about how much support you can expect from other people can be very important as you decide what to do about an unplanned pregnancy.

Part Three
Staying Healthy During Your Pregnancy

Chapter 13
Having A Healthy Pregnancy

If you've decided to have a baby, the most important thing you can do is to take good care of yourself so you and your baby will be healthy. Girls who get the proper care and make the right choices have a very good chance of having healthy babies.

Prenatal Care

See a doctor as soon as possible after you find out you're pregnant to begin getting prenatal care (prenatal care is medical care during pregnancy). The sooner you start to get medical care, the better the chances that you and your baby will be healthy.

If you can't afford to go to a doctor or clinic for prenatal care, social service organizations can help you. Ask a trusted adult, like a parent or school counselor, to help you find low-cost or free care in your community.

During your first visit, the doctor will ask you lots of questions, including the date of your last period. This helps the doctor work out how long you have been pregnant and your due date.

A baby's due date is only an estimate. In fact, women don't usually deliver exactly on their due dates. Most babies are born between 38 and 42 weeks after the first day of a woman's last period, or 36 to 40 weeks after conception (when the sperm fertilizes the egg).

Timelines

A pregnancy is divided into three phases called trimesters. The first trimester is from conception to the end of week 13. The second trimester is from week 14 to the end of week 26. The third trimester is from week 27 to the end of the pregnancy.

About This Chapter: Text in this chapter is © 1995–2017. The Nemours Foundation/KidsHealth®. Reprinted with permission.

The doctor will examine you and do a pelvic exam. Your doctor may also do blood tests, a urine test, and tests for sexually transmitted diseases (STDs). Doctors do this because some STDs can cause serious medical problems in newborns, so it's important to get treatment to protect the baby.

The doctor will probably recommend that you get some immunizations, like a Tdap vaccine to protect your baby against pertussis (whooping cough).

Your doctor will explain the types of physical and emotional changes you can expect during pregnancy. He or she will also teach you to how to recognize the signs of possible problems during pregnancy (you might hear your doctor call problems "complications"). Teens are more at risk for certain problems during pregnancy, such as anemia, high blood pressure, and giving birth earlier than usual (called premature delivery).

Your doctor will want you to start taking prenatal vitamins that contain folic acid, calcium, and iron as soon as possible. The doctor may prescribe the vitamins or recommend a brand that you can buy over-the-counter. These vitamins and minerals help ensure the baby's and mother's health as well as prevent some types of birth defects.

Ideally, you should see your doctor once each month for the first 28 weeks of your pregnancy, then every 2 weeks until 36 weeks, then once a week until you deliver the baby. If you have a medical condition such as diabetes that needs careful monitoring during your pregnancy, your doctor will probably want to see you more often.

During visits, your doctor or nurse will check your weight, blood pressure, and urine. The doctor or nurse will measure your abdomen to keep track of the baby's growth. After the baby's heartbeat can be heard with a special device, the doctor will listen for it at each visit. Your doctor will probably also send you for some other tests during the pregnancy, such as an ultrasound, to make sure that everything is OK with your baby.

One part of prenatal care is attending classes where moms to be can learn about having a healthy pregnancy and delivery. You can also learn the basics of caring for a new baby. These classes may be offered at hospitals, medical centers, schools, and colleges in your area.

It can be difficult for adults to talk to their doctors about their bodies and even more difficult for teens to do so. Your doctor is there to help you stay healthy during pregnancy and have a healthy baby—and there's probably not much he or she hasn't heard! So don't be afraid to ask questions.

Be frank when your doctor asks questions, even if they seem embarrassing. A lot of the issues the doctor brings up could affect your baby's health. Think of your doctor not just as someone who can help, but also as someone you can confide in about what's happening to you.

Changes To Expect In Your Body

Pregnancy causes lots of physical changes in the body. Here are some common ones:

Breast Growth

An increase in breast size is one of the first signs of pregnancy, and the breasts may continue to grow throughout the pregnancy. You may go up several bra sizes during the course of your pregnancy.

Skin Changes

Don't be surprised if people tell you your skin is "glowing" when you are pregnant—pregnancy causes an increase in blood volume, which can make your cheeks a little pinker than usual. And hormonal changes increase oil gland secretion, which can give your skin a shinier appearance. Acne is also common during pregnancy for the same reason.

Other skin changes caused by pregnancy hormones may include brownish or yellowish patches on the face called chloasma and a dark line on the midline of the lower abdomen, known as the linea nigra.

Also, moles or freckles that you had prior to pregnancy may become bigger and darker. Even the areola, the area around the nipples, becomes darker. Stretch marks are thin pink or purplish lines that can appear on your abdomen, breasts, or thighs.

Except for the darkening of the areola, which can last, these skin changes will usually disappear after you give birth.

Mood Swings

It's very common to have mood swings during pregnancy. Some girls may also experience depression during pregnancy or after delivery. If you have symptoms of depression such as sadness, changes in sleep patterns, thoughts of hurting yourself, or bad feelings about yourself or your life, tell your doctor so he or she can help you to get treatment.

Pregnancy Discomforts

Pregnancy can cause some uncomfortable side effects. These include:

- nausea and vomiting (especially early in the pregnancy)
- leg swelling
- varicose veins in the legs and the area around the vaginal opening

- hemorrhoids

- heartburn and constipation

- backache

- fatigue

- sleep loss

If you have one or more of these side effects, keep in mind that you're not alone! Ask your doctor for advice on how to deal with these common problems.

If you are pregnant and have bleeding or pain, call the doctor immediately, even if you are not planning to continue the pregnancy.

Things To Avoid

Smoking, drinking alcohol, and taking drugs when you are pregnant put you and your baby at risk for a number of serious problems.

Alcohol

Doctors now believe that it's not safe to drink any amount of alcohol when you are pregnant. Drinking can harm a developing fetus, putting a baby at risk for birth defects and mental problems.

Smoking

When a woman smokes while she is pregnant, she can have a miscarriage or stillbirth. Her baby might be premature (born early), and sudden infant death syndrome (SIDS).

SIDS is the sudden, unexplained death of an infant who is younger than 1 year old.

Drugs

Using drugs such as cocaine or marijuana during pregnancy can cause miscarriage, prematurity, and other medical problems. Babies can also be born addicted to some drugs.

Ask your doctor for help if you are having trouble quitting smoking, drinking, or drugs. Check with your doctor before taking any medication while you are pregnant, including over-the-counter medications, herbal remedies and supplements, and vitamins.

Unsafe Sex

Talk to your doctor about sex during pregnancy. If your doctor says it's OK to have sex while you're pregnant, you must use a condom to help prevent getting an STD. Some STDs can cause blindness, pneumonia, or meningitis in newborns, so it's important to protect yourself and your baby.

Taking Care Of Yourself During Pregnancy

Eating

Many girls worry about how their bodies look and are afraid to gain weight during pregnancy. But now that you are eating for two, this is not a good time to cut calories or go on a diet. Both you and your baby need certain nutrients so the baby can grow properly. Eating a variety of healthy foods, drinking plenty of water, and cutting back on high-fat junk foods will help you and your developing baby to be healthy.

Doctors generally recommend adding about 300 calories a day to your diet to provide adequate nourishment for the developing fetus. You should gain about 25 to 35 pounds during pregnancy, most of this during the last 6 months—although how much a girl should gain depends on how much she weighed before the pregnancy. Your doctor will advise you based on your individual situation.

Eating additional fiber—25 to 30 grams a day—and drinking plenty of water can help to prevent common problems such as constipation. Good sources of fiber are fresh fruits and vegetables and breads, cereals, or muffins that have lots of whole grain in them.

You'll need to avoid eating or drinking certain things during pregnancy, such as:

- certain types of fish, such as swordfish, canned tuna, and other fish that may be high in mercury (your doctor can help you decide which fish you can eat)

- foods that contain raw eggs, such as mousse or Caesar salad

- raw or undercooked meat and fish

- processed meats, such as hot dogs and deli meats

- soft, unpasteurized cheeses, such as feta, brie, blue, and goat cheese

- unpasteurized milk, juice, or cider

It's also a good idea to limit food or drinks that contain caffeine and artificial sweeteners.

Exercise

Exercising during pregnancy is good for you as long as you are having an uncomplicated pregnancy and choose appropriate activities. Doctors generally recommend low-impact activities such as walking, swimming, and yoga.

> Contact sports and high-impact aerobic activities that pose a greater risk of injury should generally be avoided.
>
> Also, working at a job that involves heavy lifting is not recommended for women during pregnancy.

Talk to your doctor if you have questions about whether particular types of exercise are safe for you and your baby.

Sleep

It's important to get plenty of rest while you are pregnant. Early in your pregnancy, try to get into the habit of sleeping on your side. Lying on your side with your knees bent is likely to be the most comfortable position as your pregnancy progresses. Also, it makes your heart's job easier because it keeps the baby's weight from applying pressure to the large vein that carries blood back to the heart from your feet and legs.

Some doctors recommend that girls who are pregnant sleep on the left side. Because of where some of your major blood vessels are, lying on your left side helps keep the uterus from pressing on them. Ask what your doctor recommends—in most cases, lying on either side should do the trick and help take some pressure off your back.

Throughout your pregnancy, but especially toward the end, you may wake up often at night to go to the bathroom. While it's important to drink enough water while you're pregnant, try to drink most of it during the day rather than at night. Use the bathroom right before going to bed.

As you get further along in your pregnancy, you might have a difficult time getting comfortable in bed. Try positioning pillows around and under your belly, back, or legs to get more comfortable.

Stress can also interfere with sleep. Maybe you're worried about your baby's health, about delivery, or about what your new role as a parent will be like. All of these feelings are normal, but they may keep you up at night. Talk to your doctor if you are having problems sleeping during your pregnancy.

Emotional Health

It's common for pregnant teens to feel a range of emotions, such as fear, anger, guilt, confusion, and sadness. It may take a while to adjust to the fact that you're going to have a baby. It's a huge change, and it's natural for pregnant teens to wonder whether they're ready to handle the responsibilities that come with being a parent.

How a girl feels often depends on how much support she has from the baby's father, from her family (and the baby's father's family), and from friends. Each girl's situation is different. Depending on your situation, you may need to seek more support from people outside your family. It's important to talk to the people who can support and guide you and help you share and sort through your feelings. Your school counselor or nurse can refer you to resources in your community that can help.

Sometimes girls who are pregnant have miscarriages and lose the pregnancy. This can be very upsetting and difficult to go through for some girls, although it may bring feelings of relief for others. It is important to talk about these feelings and to get support from friends and family—or if that's not possible, from people such as counselors or teachers.

School And The Future

Some girls plan to raise their babies themselves. Sometimes grandparents or other family members help. Some girls decide to give their babies up for adoption. It takes a great deal of courage and concern for the baby to make these difficult decisions.

Girls who complete high school are more likely to have good jobs and enjoy more success in their lives. If possible, finish high school now rather than trying to return later. Ask your school counselor or an adult you trust for information about programs and classes in your community for pregnant teens.

Some communities have support groups especially for teen parents. Some high schools have child-care centers on campus. Perhaps a family member or friend can care for your baby while you're in school.

You can learn more about what to expect in becoming a parent by reading books, attending classes, or checking out reputable websites on child raising. Your baby's doctor, your parents, family members, or other adults can all help guide you while you are pregnant and after the baby is born.

Chapter 14
Prenatal Care And Tests

What Is Prenatal Care?

Prenatal care is the healthcare you get while you are pregnant. Take care of yourself and your baby by:

- Getting **early** prenatal care. If you know you're pregnant, or think you might be, call your doctor to schedule a visit.

- Getting **regular** prenatal care. Your doctor will schedule you for many checkups over the course of your pregnancy. Don't miss any—they are all important.

- Following your doctor's advice.

Why Do I Need Prenatal Care?

Prenatal care can help keep you and your baby healthy. Babies of mothers who do not get prenatal care are three times more likely to have a low birth weight and five times more likely to die than those born to mothers who do get care.

Doctors can spot health problems early when they see mothers regularly. This allows doctors to treat them early. Early treatment can cure many problems and prevent others. Doctors also can talk to pregnant women about things they can do to give their unborn babies a healthy start to life.

About This Chapter: This chapter includes text excerpted from "Prenatal Care Fact Sheet," Office on Women's Health (OWH), U.S. Department of Health and Human Services (HHS), September 27, 2012. Reviewed March 2017.

I Am Thinking About Getting Pregnant. How Can I Take Care Of Myself?

You should start taking care of yourself *before* you start trying to get pregnant. This is called preconception health. It means knowing how health conditions and risk factors could affect you or your unborn baby if you become pregnant. For example, some foods, habits, and medicines can harm your baby—even before he or she is conceived. Some health problems also can affect pregnancy.

Talk to your doctor before pregnancy to learn what you can do to prepare your body. Women should prepare for pregnancy before becoming sexually active. Ideally, women should give themselves at least 3 months to prepare before getting pregnant.

The five most important things you can do before becoming pregnant are:

1. Take 400 to 800 micrograms (400 to 800 mcg or 0.4 to 0.8 mg) of folic acid every day for at least 3 months before getting pregnant to lower your risk of some birth defects of the brain and spine. You can get folic acid from some foods. But it's hard to get all the folic acid you need from foods alone. Taking a vitamin with folic acid is the best and easiest way to be sure you're getting enough.

2. Stop smoking and drinking alcohol. Ask your doctor for help.

3. If you have a medical condition, be sure it is under control. Some conditions include asthma, diabetes, depression, high blood pressure, obesity, thyroid disease, or epilepsy. Be sure your vaccinations are up to date.

4. Talk to your doctor about any over-the-counter and prescription medicines you are using. These include dietary or herbal supplements. Some medicines are not safe during pregnancy. At the same time, stopping medicines you need also can be harmful.

5. Avoid contact with toxic substances or materials at work and at home that could be harmful. Stay away from chemicals and cat or rodent feces.

I'm Pregnant. What Should I Do—Or Not Do—To Take Care Of Myself And My Unborn Baby?

Follow these do's and don'ts to take care of yourself and the precious life growing inside you:

Healthcare Do's And Don'ts

- Get early and regular prenatal care. Whether this is your first pregnancy or third, healthcare is extremely important. Your doctor will check to make sure you and the baby are healthy at each visit. If there are any problems, early action will help you and the baby.

- Take a multivitamin or prenatal vitamin with 400 to 800 micrograms (400 to 800 mcg or 0.4 to 0.8 mg) of folic acid every day. Folic acid is most important in the early stages of pregnancy, but you should continue taking folic acid throughout pregnancy.

- Ask your doctor before stopping any medicines or starting any new medicines. Some medicines are not safe during pregnancy. Keep in mind that even over-the-counter medicines and herbal products may cause side effects or other problems. But not using medicines you need could also be harmful.

- Avoid X-rays. If you must have dental work or diagnostic tests, tell your dentist or doctor that you are pregnant so that extra care can be taken.

- Get a flu shot. Pregnant women can get very sick from the flu and may need hospital care.

Food Do's And Don'ts

- Eat a variety of healthy foods. Choose fruits, vegetables, whole grains, calcium-rich foods, and foods low in saturated fat. Also, make sure to drink plenty of fluids, especially water.

- Get all the nutrients you need each day, including iron. Getting enough iron prevents you from getting anemia, which is linked to preterm birth and low birth weight. Eating a variety of healthy foods will help you get the nutrients your baby needs. But ask your doctor if you need to take a daily prenatal vitamin or iron supplement to be sure you are getting enough.

- Protect yourself and your baby from food-borne illnesses, including toxoplasmosis and listeria. Wash fruits and vegetables before eating. Don't eat uncooked or undercooked meats or fish. Always handle, clean, cook, eat, and store foods properly.

- Don't eat fish with lots of mercury, including swordfish, king mackerel, shark, and tilefish.

Lifestyle Do's And Don'ts

- Gain a healthy amount of weight. Your doctor can tell you how much weight gain you should aim for during pregnancy.

- Don't smoke, drink alcohol, or use drugs. These can cause long-term harm or death to your baby. Ask your doctor for help quitting.

- Unless your doctor tells you not to, try to get at least 2 hours and 30 minutes of moderate-intensity aerobic activity a week. It's best to spread out your workouts throughout the week. If you worked out regularly before pregnancy, you can keep up your activity level as long as your health doesn't change and you talk to your doctor about your activity level throughout your pregnancy.

- Don't take very hot baths or use hot tubs or saunas.

- Get plenty of sleep and find ways to control stress.

- Get informed. Read books, watch videos, go to a childbirth class, and talk with moms you know.

- Ask your doctor about childbirth education classes for you and your partner. Classes can help you prepare for the birth of your baby.

Environmental Do's And Don'ts

- Stay away from chemicals like insecticides, solvents (like some cleaners or paint thinners), lead, mercury, and paint (including paint fumes). Not all products have pregnancy warnings on their labels. If you're unsure if a product is safe, ask your doctor before using it. Talk to your doctor if you are worried that chemicals used in your workplace might be harmful.

- If you have a cat, ask your doctor about toxoplasmosis. This infection is caused by a parasite sometimes found in cat feces. If not treated toxoplasmosis can cause birth defects. You can lower your risk of by avoiding cat litter and wearing gloves when gardening.

- Avoid contact with rodents, including pet rodents, and with their urine, droppings, or nesting material. Rodents can carry a virus that can be harmful or even deadly to your unborn baby.

- Take steps to avoid illness, such as washing hands frequently.

- Stay away from secondhand smoke.

I Don't Want To Get Pregnant Right Now. But Should I Still Take Folic Acid Every Day?

Yes! Birth defects of the brain and spine happen in the very early stages of pregnancy, often before a woman knows she is pregnant. By the time she finds out she is pregnant, it might be too late to prevent those birth defects. Also, half of all pregnancies in the United States are not planned. For these reasons, all women who are able to get pregnant need 400 to 800 mcg of folic acid every day.

How Often Should I See My Doctor During Pregnancy?

Your doctor will give you a schedule of all the doctor's visits you should have while pregnant. Most experts suggest you see your doctor:

- About once each month for weeks 4 through 28
- Twice a month for weeks 28 through 36
- Weekly for weeks 36 to birth

If you are older than 35 or your pregnancy is high risk, you'll probably see your doctor more often.

What Happens During Prenatal Visits?

During the first prenatal visit, you can expect your doctor to:

- Ask about your health history including diseases, operations, or prior pregnancies.
- Ask about your family's health history.
- Do a complete physical exam, including a pelvic exam and Pap test.
- Take your blood and urine for lab work.
- Check your blood pressure, height, and weight.
- Calculate your due date.
- Answer your questions.

At the first visit, you should ask questions and discuss any issues related to your pregnancy. Find out all you can about how to stay healthy.

Later prenatal visits will probably be shorter. Your doctor will check on your health and make sure the baby is growing as expected. Most prenatal visits will include:

- Checking your blood pressure.
- Measuring your weight gain.

- Measuring your abdomen to check your baby's growth (once you begin to show).

- Checking the baby's heart rate.

While you're pregnant, you also will have some routine tests. Some tests are suggested for all women, such as blood work to check for anemia, your blood type, human immunodeficiency virus (HIV), and other factors. Other tests might be offered based on your age, personal or family health history, your ethnic background, or the results of routine tests you have had.

Paying For Prenatal Care

Pregnancy can be stressful if you are worried about affording healthcare for you and your unborn baby. For many women, the extra expenses of prenatal care and preparing for the new baby are overwhelming. The good news is that women in every state can get help to pay for medical care during their pregnancies. Every state in the United States has a program to help. Programs give medical care, information, advice, and other services important for a healthy pregnancy.

You may find help through these places:

- Local hospital or social service agencies–Ask to speak with a social worker on staff. She or he will be able to tell you where to go for help.
- Community clinics–Some areas have free clinics or clinics that provide free care to women in need.
- Women, Infants and Children (WIC) Program–This government program is available in every state. It provides help with food, nutritional counseling, and access to health services for women, infants, and children.
- Places of worship

(Source: "Prenatal Care And Tests," Office on Women's Health (OWH), U.S. Department of Health and Human Services (HHS).)

Where Can I Go To Get Free Or Reduced-Cost Prenatal Care?

Women in every state can get help to pay for medical care during their pregnancies. This prenatal care can help you have a healthy baby. Every state in the United States has a program to help. Programs give medical care, information, advice, and other services important for a healthy pregnancy.

To find out about the program in your state:

- Call 800-311-BABY (800-311-2229). This toll-free telephone number will connect you to the Health Department in your area code.

- For information in Spanish, call 800-504-7081.

- Contact your local Health Department.

Chapter 15

Taking Vitamins With Folic Acid During Pregnancy

Facts About Folic Acid

Centers for Disease Control and Prevention (CDC) urges women to take 400 mcg of folic acid every day, starting at least one month before getting pregnant, to help prevent major birth defects of the baby's brain and spine.

What Is Folic Acid?

Folic acid is a B vitamin. Our bodies use it to make new cells. Everyone needs folic acid.

Why Folic Acid Is So Important

Folic acid is very important because it can help prevent some major birth defects of the baby's brain and spine (anencephaly and spina bifida).

How Much Folic Acid A Woman Needs

400 micrograms (mcg) every day.

When To Start Taking Folic Acid

For folic acid to help prevent some major birth defects, a woman needs to start taking it at least one month before she becomes pregnant and while she is pregnant.

About This Chapter: Text under the heading "Facts About Folic Acid" is excerpted from "Folic Acid—Facts About Folic Acid," Centers for Disease Control and Prevention (CDC), December 14, 2016; Text under the heading "Frequently Asked Questions" is excerpted from "Folic Acid: Questions And Answers," Centers for Disease Control and Prevention (CDC), May 6, 2015.

Every woman needs folic acid every day, whether she's planning to get pregnant or not, for the healthy new cells the body makes daily. Think about the skin, hair, and nails. These—and other parts of the body—make new cells each day.

How A Woman Can Get Enough Folic Acid

There are two easy ways to be sure to get enough folic acid each day:

1. **Take a vitamin that has folic acid in it every day.**

   Most multivitamins sold in the United States have the amount of folic acid women need each day. Women can also choose to take a small pill (supplement) that has only folic acid in it each day.

> Multivitamins and folic acid pills can be found at most local pharmacy, grocery, or discount stores. Check the label to be sure it contains 100% of the daily value (DV) of folic acid, which is 400 micrograms (mcg).

2. **Eat a bowl of breakfast cereal that has 100% of the DV of folic acid every day.**

   Not every cereal has this amount. Check the label on the side of the box, and look for one that has "100%" next to folic acid.

Frequently Asked Questions

Why Can't I Wait Until I'm Pregnant—Or Planning To Get Pregnant To Start Taking Folic Acid?

Birth defects of the brain and spine (anencephaly and spina bifida) happen in the first few weeks of pregnancy; often before you find out you're pregnant. By the time you realize you're pregnant, it might be too late to prevent those birth defects. Also, half of all pregnancies in the United States are unplanned.

These are two reasons why it is important for all women who can get pregnant to be sure to get 400 mcg of folic acid every day, even if they aren't planning a pregnancy any time soon.

I'm Planning To Get Pregnant This Month. Is It Too Late To Start Taking Folic Acid?

The CDC recommends women to take 400 micrograms (mcg) of folic acid every day, starting at least one month before getting pregnant. If you are trying to get pregnant this month, or planning to get pregnant soon, start taking 400 mcg of folic acid today!

Can't I Get Enough Folic Acid By Eating A Well-Balanced Healthy Diet?

It is hard to eat a diet that has all the nutrients you need every day. Even with careful planning, you might not get all the vitamins you need from your diet alone. That's why it's important to take a vitamin with folic acid every day.

I Can't Swallow Large Pills. How Can I Take A Vitamin With Folic Acid?

These days, multivitamins with folic acid come in chewable chocolate or fruit flavors, liquids, and large oval or smaller round pills.

A single serving of many breakfast cereals also has the amount of folic acid that a woman needs each day. Check the label! Look for cereals that have 100% DV of folic acid in a serving, which is 400 micrograms (mcg).

Vitamins Cost Too Much. How Can I Get The Vitamin With Folic Acid That I Need?

Many stores offer a single folic acid supplement for just pennies a day. Another good choice is a store brand multivitamin, which includes more of the vitamins a woman needs each day. Unless your doctor suggests a special type, you do not have to choose among vitamins for women or active people. A basic multivitamin meets the needs of most women.

How Can I Remember To Take A Vitamin With Folic Acid Every Day?

Make it easy to remember by taking your vitamin at the same time every day. Try taking your vitamin when you:

- Brush your teeth, OR
- Eat breakfast, OR
- Finish your shower, OR
- Brush your hair, OR

Seeing the vitamin bottle on the bathroom or kitchen counter can help you remember it, too. If you use a cell phone or personal digital assistant (PDA), you can program it to give you a daily reminder. If you have children, you can take your vitamin when they take theirs.

Today's woman is busy! You know that you should exercise, eat right, and get enough sleep. You might wonder how you can fit another thing into your day. But it only takes a few seconds to take a vitamin to get all the folic acid you need.

Are There Other Health Benefits Of Taking Folic Acid?

Folic acid might help to prevent some other birth defects, such as cleft lip and palate and some heart defects. There might also be other health benefits of taking folic acid for both women and men. More research is needed to confirm these other health benefits. All adults should take 400 micrograms (mcg) of folic acid every day.

Is It Better To Take More Than 400 mcg Of Folic Acid Every Day?

When taking supplements, more is not better. Women who can get pregnant (whether planning to or not) need just 400 mcg of folic acid daily, and they can get this amount from vitamins or fortified foods. This is in addition to eating foods rich in folate. But, your doctor might ask you to take more for certain reasons.

What Is Folate And How Is It Different From Folic Acid?

Folate and folic acid are often used interchangeably. They're different forms of the same B vitamin. Folate is found naturally in some foods, such as leafy, dark green vegetables, citrus fruits and juices, and beans.

The body does not use folate as easily as folic acid. It is difficult to eat enough foods that are high in folate each day to help prevent neural tube defects. Women who can get pregnant should consume 400 micrograms of folic acid in addition to eating a varied diet rich in natural food folate.

What Is "Synthetic" Folic Acid?

The terms, "folic acid" and "synthetic folic acid" mean the same thing. They both refer to the man-made form of the B vitamin folate that is added to vitamins and some foods. In the United States, foods labeled as "enriched," such as bread, pasta, rice, and some breakfast cereals, have been fortified with folic acid.

Chapter 16
The Stages Of Pregnancy

What Is Pregnancy?

Pregnancy is the term used to describe the period in which a woman carries a fetus inside of her. In most cases, the fetus grows in the uterus.

(Source: "Pregnancy: Condition Information," Eunice Kennedy Shriver *National Institute of Child Health and Human Development (NICHD).)*

Pregnancy lasts about 40 weeks, counting from the first day of your last normal period. The weeks are grouped into three trimesters. Find out what's happening with you and your baby in these three stages.

First Trimester (Week 1–Week 12)

During the first trimester your body undergoes many changes. Hormonal changes affect almost every organ system in your body. These changes can trigger symptoms even in the very first weeks of pregnancy. Your period stopping is a clear sign that you are pregnant. Other changes may include:

- Extreme tiredness

- Tender, swollen breasts. Your nipples might also stick out.

- Upset stomach with or without throwing up (morning sickness)

About This Chapter: This chapter includes text excerpted from "Stages Of Pregnancy," Office on Women's Health (OWH), U.S. Department of Health and Human Services (HHS), September 27, 2010. Reviewed March 2017.

- Cravings or distaste for certain foods

- Mood swings

- Constipation (trouble having bowel movements)

- Need to pass urine more often

- Headache

- Heartburn

- Weight gain or loss

As your body changes, you might need to make changes to your daily routine, such as going to bed earlier or eating frequent, small meals. Fortunately, most of these discomforts will go away as your pregnancy progresses. And some women might not feel any discomfort at all! If you have been pregnant before, you might feel differently this time around. Just as each woman is different, so is each pregnancy.

Second Trimester (Week 13–Week 28)

Most women find the second trimester of pregnancy easier than the first. But it is just as important to stay informed about your pregnancy during these months.

You might notice that symptoms like nausea and fatigue are going away. But other new, more noticeable changes to your body are now happening. Your abdomen will expand as the baby continues to grow. And before this trimester is over, you will feel your baby beginning to move!

As your body changes to make room for your growing baby, you may have:

- Body aches, such as back, abdomen, groin, or thigh pain

- Stretch marks on your abdomen, breasts, thighs, or buttocks

- Darkening of the skin around your nipples

- A line on the skin running from belly button to pubic hairline

- Patches of darker skin, usually over the cheeks, forehead, nose, or upper lip. Patches often match on both sides of the face. This is sometimes called the mask of pregnancy.

- Numb or tingling hands, called carpal tunnel syndrome

- Itching on the abdomen, palms, and soles of the feet. (Call your doctor if you have nausea, loss of appetite, vomiting, jaundice or fatigue combined with itching. These can be signs of a serious liver problem.)

- Swelling of the ankles, fingers, and face. (If you notice any sudden or extreme swelling or if you gain a lot of weight really quickly, call your doctor right away. This could be a sign of preeclampsia.)

Third Trimester (Week 29–Week 40)

You're in the home stretch! Some of the same discomforts you had in your second trimester will continue. Plus, many women find breathing difficult and notice they have to go to the bathroom even more often. This is because the baby is getting bigger and it is putting more pressure on your organs. Don't worry, your baby is fine and these problems will lessen once you give birth.

Some new body changes you might notice in the third trimester include:

- Shortness of breath

- Heartburn

- Swelling of the ankles, fingers, and face. (If you notice any sudden or extreme swelling or if you gain a lot of weight really quickly, call your doctor right away. This could be a sign of preeclampsia.)

- Hemorrhoids

- Tender breasts, which may leak a watery pre-milk called colostrum

- Your belly button may stick out

- Trouble sleeping

- The baby "dropping," or moving lower in your abdomen

- Contractions, which can be a sign of real or false labor

As you near your due date, your cervix becomes thinner and softer (called effacing). This is a normal, natural process that helps the birth canal (vagina) to open during the birthing process. Your doctor will check your progress with a vaginal exam as you near your due date. Get excited—the final countdown has begun!

Chapter 17

The Physical Changes And Discomforts Of Pregnancy

Everyone expects pregnancy to bring an expanding waistline. But many women are surprised by the other body changes that pop up. Get the low-down on stretch marks, weight gain, heartburn and other "joys" of pregnancy. Find out what you can do to feel better.

Body Aches

As your uterus expands, you may feel aches and pains in the back, abdomen, groin area, and thighs. Many women also have backaches and aching near the pelvic bone due the pressure of the baby's head, increased weight, and loosening joints. Some pregnant women complain of pain that runs from the lower back, down the back of one leg, to the knee or foot. This is called sciatica. It is thought to occur when the uterus puts pressure on the sciatic nerve.

What might help:

- Lie down.

- Rest.

- Apply heat.

Call the doctor if pain does not get better.

About This Chapter: This chapter includes text excerpted from "Body Changes And Discomforts," Office on Women's Health (OWH), U.S. Department of Health and Human Services (HHS), September 27, 2010. Reviewed March 2017.

Breast Changes

A woman's breasts increase in size and fullness during pregnancy. As the due date approaches, hormone changes will cause your breasts to get even bigger to prepare for breastfeeding. Your breasts may feel full, heavy, or tender.

In the third trimester, some pregnant women begin to leak colostrum from their breasts. Colostrum is the first milk that your breasts produce for the baby. It is a thick, yellowish fluid containing antibodies that protect newborns from infection.

What might help:

- Wear a maternity bra with good support.

- Put pads in bra to absorb leakage.

Tell your doctor if you feel a lump or have nipple changes or discharge (that is not colostrum) or skin changes.

Constipation

Many pregnant women complain of constipation. Signs of constipation include having hard, dry stools; fewer than three bowel movements per week; and painful bowel movements.

Higher levels of hormones due to pregnancy slow down digestion and relax muscles in the bowels leaving many women constipated. Plus, the pressure of the expanding uterus on the bowels can contribute to constipation.

What might help:

- Drink eight to 10 glasses of water daily.

- Don't drink caffeine.

- Eat fiber-rich foods, such as fresh or dried fruit, raw vegetables, and whole-grain cereals and breads.

- Try mild physical activity.

Tell your doctor if constipation does not go away.

Dizziness

Many pregnant women complain of dizziness and lightheadedness throughout their pregnancies. Fainting is rare but does happen even in some healthy pregnant women. There are many reasons for these symptoms. The growth of more blood vessels in early pregnancy, the pressure of the expanding uterus on blood vessels, and the body's increased need for food all can make a pregnant woman feel lightheaded and dizzy.

What might help:

- Stand up slowly.
- Avoid standing for too long.
- Don't skip meals.
- Lie on your left side.
- Wear loose clothing.

Call your doctor if you feel faint and have vaginal bleeding or abdominal pain.

Fatigue And Sleep Problems

During your pregnancy, you might feel tired even after you've had a lot of sleep. Many women find they're exhausted in the first trimester. Don't worry, this is normal! This is your body's way of telling you that you need more rest. In the second trimester, tiredness is usually replaced with a feeling of well being and energy. But in the third trimester, exhaustion often sets in again. As you get larger, sleeping may become more difficult. The baby's movements, bathroom runs, and an increase in the body's metabolism might interrupt or disturb your sleep. Leg cramping can also interfere with a good night's sleep.

What might help:

- Lie on your left side.
- Use pillows for support, such as behind your back, tucked between your knees, and under your tummy.
- Practice good sleep habits, such as going to bed and getting up at the same time each day and using your bed only for sleep and sex.
- Go to bed a little earlier.
- Nap if you are not able to get enough sleep at night.
- Drink needed fluids earlier in the day, so you can drink less in the hours before bed.

Heartburn And Indigestion

Hormones and the pressure of the growing uterus cause indigestion and heartburn. Pregnancy hormones slow down the muscles of the digestive tract. So food tends to move more slowly and digestion is sluggish. This causes many pregnant women to feel bloated.

Hormones also relax the valve that separates the esophagus from the stomach. This allows food and acids to come back up from the stomach to the esophagus. The food and acid causes the burning feeling of heartburn. As your baby gets bigger, the uterus pushes on the stomach making heartburn more common in later pregnancy.

What might help:

- Eat several small meals instead of three large meals—eat slowly.

- Drink fluids between meals—not with meals.

- Don't eat greasy and fried foods.

- Avoid citrus fruits or juices and spicy foods.

- Do not eat or drink within a few hours of bedtime.

- Do not lie down right after meals.

Call your doctor if symptoms don't improve after trying these suggestions. Ask your doctor about using an antacid.

Hemorrhoids

Hemorrhoids are swollen and bulging veins in the rectum. They can cause itching, pain, and bleeding. Up to 50 percent of pregnant women get hemorrhoids. Hemorrhoids are common during pregnancy for many reasons. During pregnancy blood volume increases greatly, which can cause veins to enlarge. The expanding uterus also puts pressure on the veins in the rectum. Plus, constipation can worsen hemorrhoids. Hemorrhoids usually improve after delivery.

What might help:

- Drink lots of fluids.

- Eat fiber-rich foods, like whole grains, raw or cooked leafy green vegetables, and fruits.

- Try not to strain with bowel movements.

- Talk to your doctor about using products such as witch hazel to soothe hemorrhoids.

Itching

About 20 percent of pregnant women feel itchy during pregnancy. Usually women feel itchy in the abdomen. But red, itchy palms and soles of the feet are also common complaints. Pregnancy hormones and stretching skin are probably to blame for most of your discomfort. Usually the itchy feeling goes away after delivery.

What might help:

- Use gentle soaps and moisturizing creams.

- Avoid hot showers and baths.

- Avoid itchy fabrics.

Call your doctor if symptoms don't improve after a week of self-care.

Leg Cramps

At different times during your pregnancy, you might have sudden muscle spasms in your legs or feet. They usually occur at night. This is due to a change in the way your body processes calcium.

What might help:

- Gently stretch muscles.

- Get mild exercise.

- For sudden cramps, flex your foot forward.

- Eat calcium-rich foods.

- Ask your doctor about calcium supplements.

Morning Sickness

In the first trimester hormone changes can cause nausea and vomiting. This is called "morning sickness," although it can occur at any time of day. Morning sickness usually tapers off by the second trimester.

What might help:

- Eat several small meals instead of three large meals to keep your stomach from being empty.

- Don't lie down after meals.

- Eat dry toast, saltines, or dry cereals before getting out of bed in the morning.

- Eat bland foods that are low in fat and easy to digest, such as cereal, rice, and bananas.

- Sip on water, weak tea, or clear soft drinks. Or eat ice chips.

- Avoid smells that upset your stomach.

Call your doctor if you have flu-like symptoms, which may signal a more serious condition.

Call your doctor if you have severe, constant nausea and/or vomiting several times every day.

Nasal Problems

Nosebleeds and nasal stuffiness are common during pregnancy. They are caused by the increased amount of blood in your body and hormones acting on the tissues of your nose.

What might help:

- Blow your nose gently.

- Drink fluids and use a cool mist humidifier.

- To stop a nosebleed, squeeze your nose between your thumb and forefinger for a few minutes.

Call your doctor if nosebleeds are frequent and do not stop after a few minutes.

Numb Or Tingling Hands

Feelings of swelling, tingling, and numbness in fingers and hands, called carpal tunnel syndrome, can occur during pregnancy. These symptoms are due to swelling of tissues in the narrow passages in your wrists, and they should disappear after delivery.

What might help:

- Take frequent breaks to rest hands.

- Ask your doctor about fitting you for a splint to keep wrists straight.

Stretch Marks And Skin Changes

Stretch marks are red, pink, or brown streaks on the skin. Most often they appear on the thighs, buttocks, abdomen, and breasts. These scars are caused by the stretching of the skin, and usually appear in the second half of pregnancy.

Some women notice other skin changes during pregnancy. For many women, the nipples become darker and browner during pregnancy. Many pregnant women also develop a dark line (called the linea nigra) on the skin that runs from the bellybutton down to the pubic hairline. Patches of darker skin usually over the cheeks, forehead, nose, or upper lip also are common. Patches often match on both sides of the face. These spots are called melasma or chloasma and are more common in darker-skinned women.

What might help:

- Be patient—stretch marks and other changes usually fade after delivery.

Swelling

Many women develop mild swelling in the face, hands, or ankles at some point in their pregnancies. As the due date approaches, swelling often becomes more noticeable.

What might help:

- Drink eight to 10 glasses of fluids daily.
- Don't drink caffeine or eat salty foods.
- Rest and elevate your feet.
- Ask your doctor about support hose.

Call your doctor if your hands or feet swell suddenly or you rapidly gain weight—it may be preeclampsia.

Urinary Frequency And Leaking

Temporary bladder control problems are common in pregnancy. Your unborn baby pushes down on the bladder, urethra, and pelvic floor muscles. This pressure can lead to more frequent need to urinate, as well as leaking of urine when sneezing, coughing, or laughing.

What might help:

- Take frequent bathroom breaks.
- Drink plenty of fluids to avoid dehydration.
- Do Kegel exercises to tone pelvic muscles.

Call your doctor if you experience burning along with frequency of urination—it may be an infection.

Varicose Veins

During pregnancy, blood volume increases greatly. This can cause veins to enlarge. Plus, pressure on the large veins behind the uterus causes the blood to slow in its return to the heart. For these reasons, varicose veins in the legs and anus (hemorrhoids) are more common in pregnancy.

Varicose veins look like swollen veins raised above the surface of the skin. They can be twisted or bulging and are dark purple or blue in color. They are found most often on the backs of the calves or on the inside of the leg.

What might help:

- Avoid tight knee-highs.

- Sit with your legs and feet raised.

Chapter 18
Nutrition And Exercise During Pregnancy

Healthy Eating

How Much Should I Eat?

Eating healthy foods and the right amount of calories helps you and your baby gain the proper amount of weight.

How much food you need depends on things like your weight before pregnancy, your age, and how fast you gain weight. In the first 3 months of pregnancy, most women do not need extra calories. You also may not need extra calories during the final weeks of pregnancy.

Check with your doctor about this. If you are not gaining the right amount of weight, your doctor may advise you to eat more calories. If you are gaining too much weight, you may need to cut down on calories. Each woman's needs are different. Your needs depend on if you were underweight, overweight, or obese before you became pregnant, or if you are having more than one baby.

What Kinds Of Foods Should I Eat?

A healthy eating plan for pregnancy includes nutrient-rich foods. Current U.S. dietary guidelines advise eating these foods each day:

- fruits and veggies (provide vitamins and fiber)

- whole grains, like oatmeal, whole-wheat bread, and brown rice (provide fiber, B vitamins, and other needed nutrients)

About This Chapter: This chapter includes text excerpted from "Health Tips For Pregnant Women," National Institute of Diabetes and Digestive and Kidney Diseases (NIDDK), June 2013. Reviewed March 2017.

Gaining The Recommended Amount Of Weight During Pregnancy

Gaining less than the recommended amount of weight in pregnancy is associated with delivering a baby who is too small. Some babies born too small may have difficulty starting breastfeeding, may be at increased risk for illness, and may experience developmental delays (not meeting the milestones for his or her age).

Gaining more than the recommended amount of weight in pregnancy is associated with having a baby who is born too large, which can lead to delivery complications, Cesarean delivery, and obesity during childhood. Gaining more than the recommended amount of weight can also increase the amount of weight you hold on to after pregnancy, which can lead to obesity.

(Source: "Weight Gain During Pregnancy," Centers for Disease Control and Prevention (CDC).)

- fat-free or low-fat milk and milk products or non-dairy soy, almond, rice, or other drinks with added calcium and vitamin D

- protein from healthy sources, like beans and peas, eggs, lean meats, seafood (8 to 12 ounces per week), and unsalted nuts and seeds

A healthy eating plan also limits salt, solid fats (like butter, lard, and shortening), and sugar-sweetened drinks and foods.

Does your eating plan measure up? How can you improve your eating habits? Try eating fruit like berries or a banana with low-fat yogurt for breakfast, a salad with beans for lunch, and a lean chicken breast and steamed veggies for dinner. Think about things you can try.

What If I Am A Vegetarian

A vegetarian eating plan during pregnancy can be healthy. Talk to your healthcare provider to make sure you are getting calcium, iron, protein, vitamin B12, vitamin D, and other needed nutrients. He or she may ask you to meet with a registered dietitian (a nutrition expert who has a degree in diet and nutrition approved by the Academy of Nutrition and Dietetics, has passed a national exam, and is licensed to practice in your state) who can help you plan meals. Your doctor may also tell you to take vitamins and minerals that will help you meet your needs.

Do I Have Any Special Nutrition Needs Now That I Am Pregnant?

Yes. During pregnancy, you need more vitamins and minerals, like folate, iron, and calcium.

Getting the right amount of folate is very important. Folate, a B vitamin also known as folic acid, may help prevent birth defects. Before pregnancy, you need 400 mcg per day. During pregnancy and when breastfeeding, you need 600 mcg per day from foods or vitamins. Foods high in folate include orange juice, strawberries, spinach, broccoli, beans, and fortified breads and breakfast cereals.

Most healthcare providers tell women who are pregnant to take a prenatal vitamin every day and eat a healthy diet. Ask your doctor about what you should take.

What Other New Eating Habits May Help My Weight Gain?

Pregnancy can create some new food and eating concerns. Meet the needs of your body and be more comfortable with these tips:

- **Eat breakfast every day.** If you feel sick to your stomach in the morning, try dry whole-wheat toast or whole-grain crackers when you first wake up. Eat them even before you get out of bed. Eat the rest of your breakfast (fruit, oatmeal, whole-grain cereal, low-fat milk or yogurt, or other foods) later in the morning.

- **Eat high-fiber foods.** Eating high-fiber foods, drinking plenty of water, and getting daily physical activity may help prevent constipation. Try to eat whole-grain cereals, vegetables, fruits, and beans.

- **If you have heartburn, eat small meals more often.** Try to eat slowly and avoid spicy and fatty foods (such as hot peppers or fried chicken). Have drinks between meals instead of with meals. Do not lie down soon after eating.

What Foods Should I Avoid?

There are certain foods and drinks that can harm your baby if you have them while you are pregnant. Here is a list of items you should avoid:

- **Alcohol.** Do not drink alcohol like wine or beer. Enjoy decaf coffee or tea, non-sugar-sweetened drinks, or water with a dash of juice. Avoid diet drinks and drinks with caffeine.

- **Fish that may have high levels of mercury** (a substance that can build up in fish and harm an unborn baby). You should eat 8 to 12 ounces of seafood per week, but limit white (albacore) tuna to 6 ounces per week. Do not eat tilefish, shark, swordfish, and king mackerel.

- **Anything that is not food.** Some pregnant women may crave something that is not food, such as laundry starch or clay. This may mean that you are not getting the right amount of a nutrient. Talk to your doctor if you crave something that is not food. He or she can help you get the right amount of nutrients.

Physical Activity

Almost all women can and should be physically active during pregnancy. Regular physical activity may

- help you and your baby gain the right amounts of weight
- reduce backaches, leg cramps, and bloating
- reduce your risk for gestational diabetes (diabetes that develops when a woman is pregnant)

If you were physically active before you became pregnant, you may not need to change your exercise habits. Talk with your healthcare provider about how to change your workouts during pregnancy.

How Much Physical Activity Do I Need?

Most women need the same amount of physical activity as before they became pregnant. Aim for at least 30 minutes of aerobic activity per day on most days of the week. Aerobic activities use large muscle groups (back, chest, and legs) to increase heart rate and breathing.

The aerobic activity should last at least 10 minutes at a time and should be of moderate intensity. This means it makes you breathe harder but does not overwork or overheat you.

If you have health issues like obesity, high blood pressure, diabetes, or anemia (too few healthy red blood cells), ask your healthcare provider about a level of activity that is safe for you.

How Can I Stay Active While Pregnant?

Even if you have not been active before, you can be active during your pregnancy by using the tips below:

- Go for a walk around the block, in a local park, or in a shopping mall with a family member or friend. If you already have children, take them with you and make it a family outing.

- Get up and move around at least once an hour if you sit in a chair most of the day. When watching TV, get up and move around during commercials. Even a simple activity like walking in place can help.

How Can I Stay Safe While Being Active?

For your health and safety, and for your baby's, you should not do some physical activities while pregnant. Some of these are listed below. Talk to your healthcare provider about other physical activities that you should not do.

Make a plan to be active while pregnant. List the activities you would like to do, such as walking or taking a prenatal yoga class. Think of the days and times you could do each activity on your list, like first thing in the morning, during lunch break from work, after dinner, or on Saturday afternoon. Look at your calendar or planner to find the days and times that work best, and commit to those plans.

Safety Do's And Dont's

Follow these safety tips while being active.

Do...

- Choose moderate activities that are not likely to injure you, such as walking or aqua aerobics.
- Drink fluids before, during, and after being physically active.
- Wear comfortable clothing that fits well and supports and protects your breasts.
- Stop exercising if you feel dizzy, short of breath, tired, or sick to your stomach.

Don't...

- Avoid brisk exercise outside during very hot weather.
- Don't use steam rooms, hot tubs, and saunas.
- After the end of week 12 of your pregnancy, avoid exercises that call for you to lie flat on your back.

Chapter 19

Weight Gain During Pregnancy

The amount of weight you gain during pregnancy is important for the health of your pregnancy and for the long-term health of you and your baby. Learn about pregnancy weight gain recommendations and steps you can take to meet your pregnancy weight gain goal.

How Much Weight Should You Gain During Pregnancy?

How much weight you should gain during pregnancy is based on your body mass index (BMI) before pregnancy. BMI is a measure of body fat calculated from weight and height.

BMI is calculated as weight ÷ height^2.

(Source: "About Child And Teen BMI," Centers for Disease Control and Prevention (CDC).)

Calculate your BMI and weight category using your weight before you became pregnant:

About This Chapter: This chapter includes text excerpted from "Weight Gain During Pregnancy," Centers for Disease Control and Prevention (CDC), October 14, 2016.

Table 19.1. Weight Gain Recommendations For Women Pregnant With One Baby

If Before Pregnancy, You Were...	You Should Gain...
Underweight BMI less than 18.5	28–40 pounds
Normal Weight BMI 18.5–24.9	25–35 pounds
Overweight BMI 25.0–29.9	15–25 pounds
Obese BMI greater than or equal to 30.0	11–20 pounds

Table 19.2. Weight Gain Recommendations For Women Pregnant With Twins

If Before Pregnancy, You Were...	You Should Gain...
Underweight BMI less than 18.5	50–62 pounds
Normal Weight BMI 18.5–24.9	37–54 pounds
Overweight BMI 25.0–29.9	31–50 pounds
Obese BMI greater than or equal to 30.0	25–42 pounds

What Percentage Of Women Are Within Pregnancy Weight Gain Recommendations?

Recent studies found that only about one-third (32%) of women gained the recommended amount of weight during pregnancy and most women gained weight outside the recommendations (21% too little, 48% too much).

Why Is It Important To Gain The Recommended Amount Of Weight During Pregnancy?

Gaining less than the recommended amount of weight in pregnancy is associated with delivering a baby who is too small. Some babies born too small may have difficulty starting breastfeeding, may be at increased risk for illness, and may experience developmental delays (not meeting the milestones for his or her age).

Gaining more than the recommended amount of weight in pregnancy is associated with having a baby who is born too large, which can lead to delivery complications, Cesarean delivery, and obesity during childhood. Gaining more than the recommended amount of weight can also increase the amount of weight you hold on to after pregnancy, which can lead to obesity.

What Steps Can You Take To Meet Pregnancy Weight Gain Recommendations?

- **Work with your healthcare provider** on your weight gain goals at the beginning and regularly throughout your pregnancy.

- **Track your pregnancy weight gain at the beginning and regularly throughout pregnancy** and compare your progress to recommended ranges of healthy weight gain.

- **Eat a balanced diet** high in whole grains, vegetables, fruits, low fat dairy, and lean protein. Use the MyPlate daily checklist (www.choosemyplate.gov/MyPlate-Daily-Checklist-input) to see the daily food group targets that are right for you at your stage of pregnancy. Most foods are safe to eat during pregnancy, but you will need to use caution with or avoid certain foods. Talk with your healthcare provider or visit Checklist of Foods to Avoid During Pregnancy (www.foodsafety.gov/risk/pregnant/chklist_pregnancy.html) for more information about food safety in pregnancy.

Table 19.3. Sample Balanced Diet Snacks For Women Who Begin Pregnancy Underweight

Sample Snacks		
1st Trimester	*No additional calories needed*	*No additional calories needed*
2nd Trimester Additional 400 calories/day	**Hardboiled egg and English muffin topped with fruit (140 calories)** • ½ of a 100% whole wheat English muffin • 1 medium strawberry, sliced • 1 large hardboiled egg **Cereal and milk (263 calories)** • 1¼ cup of high fiber cereal • 1 cup of skim milk	**Yogurt with fruit (131 calories)** • 1 6 oz. container of plain, fat free Greek yogurt • ½ cup of blackberries **Edamame, grape tomatoes, and carrots with hummus (264 calories)** • ½ cup edamame • 1 cup grape tomatoes • 4 carrot sticks • ¼ cup hummus

Table 19.3. Continued

Sample Snacks		
3rd Trimester Additional 400-600 calories/day	**Oatmeal and a glass of milk (226 calories)** • 1 cup cooked regular oatmeal, made with water • 8 oz. glass of skim milk **Crackers, peanut butter, and string cheese (267 calories)** • 5 100% whole grain crackers • 1 tablespoon of peanut butter (spread thinly on crackers) • 1 part skim string cheese stick	**Berry smoothie (211 calories)** • 1 cup of frozen unsweetened blueberries • ½ cup of skim milk • ½ cup fat free plain yogurt • 1 teaspoon honey **Apple, almonds, and cottage cheese (305 calories)** • 1 large apple, sliced • 14 almonds • ½ cup low fat cottage cheese

(Source: "Tracking Your Weight—For Women Who Begin Pregnancy Underweight," Centers for Disease Control and Prevention (CDC).)

Table 19.4. Sample Balanced Diet Snacks For Women Who Begin Pregnancy At A Normal Weight

Sample Snacks		
1st Trimester	*No additional calories needed*	*No additional calories needed*
2nd Trimester Additional 400 calories/day	**Hardboiled egg and English muffin topped with fruit (140 calories)** • ½ of a 100% whole wheat English muffin • 1 medium strawberry, sliced • 1 large hardboiled egg **Cereal and milk (263 calories)** • 1¼ cup of high fiber cereal • 1 cup of skim milk	**Yogurt with fruit (131 calories)** • 1 6 oz. container of plain, fat free Greek yogurt • ½ cup of blackberries **Edamame, grape tomatoes, and carrots with hummus (264 calories)** • ½ cup edamame • 1 cup grape tomatoes • 4 carrot sticks • ¼ cup hummus

Table 19.4. Continued

Sample Snacks		
3rd Trimester Additional 400 calories/day	**Oatmeal and a glass of milk (226 calories)** • 1 cup cooked regular oatmeal, made with water • 8 oz. glass of skim milk **Crackers and string cheese (170 calories)** • 5 100% whole grain crackers • 1 part skim string cheese stick	**Berry smoothie (211 calories)** • 1 cup of frozen unsweetened blueberries • ½ cup of skim milk • ½ cup fat free plain yogurt • 1 teaspoon honey **Apple and cottage cheese (207 calories)** • 1 large apple, sliced • ½ cup low fat cottage cheese

(Source: "Tracking Your Weight—For Women Who Begin Pregnancy At A Normal Weight," Centers for Disease Control and Prevention (CDC).)

Table 19.5. Sample Balanced Diet Snacks For Women Who Begin Pregnancy Overweight

Sample Snacks		
1st Trimester	*No additional calories needed*	*No additional calories needed*
2nd Trimester Additional 200-400 calories/day	**Hardboiled egg and fruit (100 calories)** • 1 large hardboiled egg • ½ cup strawberries **Cereal and milk (241 calories)** • 1¼ cup of high fiber cereal • 1 cup of almond milk	**Yogurt with fruit (93 calories)** • ½ cup plain Greek yogurt • ½ cup of blackberries **Edamame and carrots with hummus (215 calories)** • ½ cup edamame • 4 carrot sticks • ¼ cup hummus

Table 19.5. Continued

Sample Snacks		
3rd Trimester Additional 400 calories/day	**Oatmeal and a glass of milk (226 calories)** • 1 cup cooked regular oatmeal, made with water • 8 oz. glass of skim milk **Crackers and string cheese (170 calories)** • 5 100% whole grain crackers • 1 part skim string cheese stick	**Berry smoothie (211 calories)** • 1 cup of frozen unsweetened blueberries • ½ cup of skim milk • ½ cup fat free plain yogurt • 1 teaspoon honey **Apple and cottage cheese (207 calories)** • 1 large apple, sliced • ½ cup low fat cottage cheese

(Source: "Tracking Your Weight—For Women Who Begin Pregnancy Overweight," Centers for Disease Control and Prevention (CDC).)

Table 19.6. Sample Balanced Diet Snacks For Women Who Begin Pregnancy With Obesity

Sample Snacks		
1st Trimester	*No additional calories needed*	*No additional calories needed*
2nd Trimester Additional 200 calories/day	**Hardboiled egg and fruit (100 calories)** • 1 large hardboiled egg • ½ cup strawberries **Cereal (111 calories)** • ¾ cup dry high fiber cereal	**Yogurt with fruit (93 calories)** • ½ cup plain Greek yogurt • 1/3 cup raspberries **Edamame (95 calories)** • ½ cup edamame
3rd Trimester Additional 400 calories/day	**Oatmeal and a glass of milk (226 calories)** • 1 cup cooked regular oatmeal, made with water • 8 oz. glass of skim milk **Crackers and string cheese (170 calories)** • 5 100% whole grain crackers • 1 part skim string cheese stick	**Berry smoothie (211 calories)** • 1 cup of frozen unsweetened blueberries • ½ cup of skim milk • ½ cup fat free plain yogurt • 1 teaspoon honey **Apple and cottage cheese (207 calories)** • 1 large apple, sliced • ½ cup low fat cottage cheese

(Source: "Tracking Your Weight—For Women Who Begin Pregnancy With Obesity," Centers for Disease Control and Prevention (CDC).)

- **Limit added sugars and solid fats** found in foods like soft drinks, desserts, fried foods, whole milk, and fatty meats.

- **Know your calorie needs.** In general, the first trimester (or first three months) does not require any extra calories. Typically, women need about 340 additional calories per day during the second trimester (second three months) and about 450 additional calories per day during the third (last) trimester.

- **Work up to or maintain at least 150 minutes (2 ½ hours) of moderate intensity aerobic activity (such as brisk walking) per week.** 150 minutes may sound overwhelming, but you can achieve your goal by breaking up your physical activity into 10 minutes at a time. Physical activity is healthy and safe for most pregnant women. Talk to your healthcare provider to determine if you have any physical activity restrictions.

Chapter 20
Eating Disorders During Pregnancy

Adequate nutrition is vital during pregnancy to ensure the health and well-being of both mother and baby. As a result, pregnancy may present challenges for women who are struggling with or recovering from eating disorders. Pregnancy creates physical and emotional changes that can be stressful for anyone, but especially for women who have preexisting mental health conditions. Even women who believe they have put their disordered eating behaviors in the past may be vulnerable to relapse due to the bodily changes associated with pregnancy. The normal weight gain during pregnancy can trigger symptoms of anorexia, for instance, while the feelings of fullness as the baby grows can create an urge to purge among people with bulimia. The food cravings that often occur during pregnancy can also be problematic for people with binge eating disorder.

If left untreated during pregnancy, active eating disorders can cause serious complications that jeopardize the health of both mother and baby. Mothers with eating disorders are more likely to deliver by Cesarean section and experience postpartum depression. Meanwhile, babies born to mothers with eating disorders have a high risk of premature delivery, low birth weight, and small head circumference. On the other hand, some women find it easier to avoid disordered eating behavior during pregnancy as their focus shifts to protecting the health and welfare of the fetus. Given the importance of nutrition throughout pregnancy, however, women with eating disorders should seek professional advice and treatment to ensure that the condition does not interfere with the normal growth and development of the baby.

"Eating Disorders During Pregnancy," © 2017 Omnigraphics. Reviewed March 2017.

Recognizing The Signs Of Eating Disorders

Eating disorders may impact a woman's reproductive health even before she becomes pregnant. Women with anorexia or bulimia often experience irregularity or cessation of menstrual cycles, for instance, which can affect fertility and reduce the likelihood of conception. Therefore, doctors recommend that women bring eating disorders under control and maintain a healthy weight for several months before trying to get pregnant. Even in such cases, however, some women find that the bodily changes associated with pregnancy may trigger or exacerbate the symptoms of eating disorders. Some of the common signs that a woman is struggling with an eating disorder during pregnancy include:

- weight loss or very limited weight gain throughout the pregnancy
- anxiety about being overweight
- restricting food intake, skipping meals, or eliminating major food groups
- vomiting or purging to get rid of calories consumed
- extreme (to the point of exhaustion) or excessive exercising to stay thin
- chronic fatigue, dizziness, or fainting
- depression, lack of interest in socializing, or avoidance of family and friends

If these signs appear during pregnancy, it is important to seek treatment to ensure a healthy outcome for both mother and baby.

Understanding The Risks Of Eating Disorders

Left untreated, eating disorders can have debilitating effects on the health of both the pregnant woman and the unborn baby. Understanding the risks posed by eating disorders may encourage expectant mothers to get the help they need to have a healthy pregnancy. Some of the potential health risks for a pregnant woman with an eating disorder include:

- severe dehydration or malnutrition
- high blood pressure (preeclampsia), gestational diabetes, or anemia
- cardiac irregularities
- miscarriage, stillbirth, or premature labor
- complications during delivery and increased risk of Cesarean section
- extended time required to heal from childbirth

- postpartum depression

- difficulties breastfeeding

- low self-esteem and poor body image

- social withdrawal, isolation, and marital or family conflicts

Eating disorders also carry a number of serious risks for the developing baby, including:

- malnutrition, abnormal fetal growth, or poor development

- premature birth

- respiratory distress

- small head circumference

- low birth weight (with anorexia or bulimia)

- high birth weight (with binge eating disorder)

- feeding difficulties

The seriousness of these risks, along with the natural maternal instinct to protect the developing baby, enables some women to effectively manage their eating disorders during pregnancy.

Managing Eating Disorders In Pregnancy

For some women, on the other hand, the physical and emotional changes that occur during pregnancy may trigger or worsen eating disorder symptoms. Those with anorexia, for instance, may struggle with their inability to fully control their eating and weight gain while pregnant.

Pregnant women who are struggling with eating disorders should see a counselor or therapist to help guide them through pregnancy-related changes, fears about weight gain, and concerns about body image. In addition, they should work with a nutritionist or dietitian to learn about nutritional requirements during pregnancy, ensure that caloric intake is sufficient to support fetal development, and create appropriate meal plans. Finally, they should inform their obstetrician about their eating disorder and make regular visits to track prenatal growth. The pregnancy may be classified as "high risk" so that the healthcare provider can carefully monitor the health of both mother and baby. Additional tips to help alleviate concerns and manage eating disorders during pregnancy include:

- remember that the source of weight gain is a growing baby

- avoid the scale, and ask the healthcare provider not to share your weight during checkups

- try to ignore, or at least not dwell on, comments others make about your pregnant body

- avoid looking at magazines that feature unrealistic postnatal weight-loss stories

Maintaining Health After Childbirth

Even when women with eating disorders manage to keep them under control during pregnancy, many tend to suffer relapses following childbirth. Women face extreme social pressure to lose pregnancy weight as quickly as possible. As a result, many women feel that they must begin a weight-loss diet or exercise regimen immediately after their baby has been born. This pressure to shed pounds can trigger disordered eating behaviors. Experts recommend focusing instead on the remarkable physical accomplishment of growing and delivering a healthy baby. This focus can help women accept the changes in body shape and appearance that may have resulted from pregnancy and childbirth.

Experts also stress that it is important for women to take care of their own health following childbirth. Women with eating disorders are particularly susceptible to postnatal depression, so they should watch out for symptoms and seek professional help if they appear. Many women with eating disorders also express concerns about their ability to breastfeed. As long as the eating disorder is under control, it should not affect breastfeeding. But it is important to remember that restricting caloric intake during breastfeeding can reduce both the quantity and quality of breastmilk. Adequate nutrition is also important to ensure that new mothers have the energy, health, and well-being necessary to love, care for, and enjoy their infant.

References

1. "Eating Disorders and Pregnancy," Eating Disorder Hope, May 25, 2013.

2. "Eating Disorders and Pregnancy," Eating Disorders Victoria, June 24, 2015.

3. "Pregnancy and Eating Disorders," American Pregnancy Association, July 2015.

Chapter 21
Sleeping During Pregnancy

Expectant parents know that it'll be harder to get a good night's sleep after their little one arrives. But who could have guessed that catching enough ZZZs during pregnancy could be so difficult?

Actually, you may sleep more than usual during the first trimester of your pregnancy. It's normal to feel tired as your body works to protect and nurture the developing baby. The placenta (the organ that nourishes the fetus until birth) is just forming, your body is making more blood, and your heart is pumping faster.

It's usually later in pregnancy that most women have trouble getting enough deep, uninterrupted sleep.

Why Sleeping Can Be Difficult

The first and most pressing reason behind sleep problems during pregnancy is the increasing size of the fetus, which can make it hard to find a comfortable sleeping position. If you've always been a back or stomach sleeper, you might have trouble getting used to sleeping on your side (as doctors recommend). Also, shifting around in bed becomes more difficult as the pregnancy progresses and you get bigger.

Other common physical symptoms may interfere with sleep as well:

- **the frequent urge to pee:** Your kidneys are working harder to filter the increased volume of blood moving through your body, and this filtering process creates more urine. And,

About This Chapter: Text in this chapter is © 1995-2017. The Nemours Foundation/KidsHealth®. Reprinted with permission.

as your baby grows and the uterus gets bigger, the pressure on your bladder increases. This means more trips to the bathroom, day and night. The number of nighttime trips may be greater if your baby is particularly active at night.

- **increased heart rate:** Your heart rate increases to pump more blood, and as more of your blood supply goes to the uterus, your heart works harder to send sufficient blood to the rest of your body.

- **shortness of breath:** The increase of pregnancy hormones will cause you to breathe in more deeply. You might feel like you're working harder to get air. Later on, breathing can feel more difficult as your enlarging uterus takes up more space, resulting in pressure against your diaphragm (the muscle just below your lungs).

- **leg cramps and backaches:** The extra weight you're carrying can contribute to pains in your legs or back. During pregnancy, the body also makes a hormone called relaxin, which helps prepare it for childbirth. One of the effects of relaxin is the loosening of ligaments throughout the body, making pregnant women less stable and more prone to injury, especially in their backs.

- **heartburn and constipation:** Many pregnant women have heartburn, which is when the stomach contents reflux back up into the esophagus. During pregnancy, the entire digestive system slows down and food stays in the stomach and intestines longer, which may cause heartburn or constipation. These can both get worse later on in the pregnancy when the growing uterus presses on the stomach or the large intestine.

Your sleep problems might have other causes as well. Many pregnant women report that their dreams become more vivid than usual, and some even have nightmares.

Stress can interfere with sleep, too. Maybe you're worried about your baby's health, anxious about your abilities as a parent, or feeling nervous about the delivery itself. All of these feelings are normal, but they might keep you (and your partner) up at night.

Finding A Good Sleeping Position

Early in your pregnancy, try to get into the habit of sleeping on your side. Lying on your side with your knees bent is likely to be the most comfortable position as your pregnancy progresses. It also makes your heart's job easier because it keeps the baby's weight from applying pressure to the large vein (called the inferior vena cava) that carries blood back to the heart from your feet and legs.

Some doctors specifically recommend that pregnant women sleep on the **left side**. Because your liver is on the right side of your abdomen, lying on your left side helps keep the uterus off that large organ. Sleeping on the left side also improves circulation to the heart and allows for the best blood flow to the fetus, uterus, and kidneys. Ask your doctor what he or she recommends.

But don't drive yourself crazy worrying that you might roll over onto your back during the night. Shifting positions is a natural part of sleeping that you can't control. Most likely, during the third trimester of your pregnancy, your body won't shift into the back-sleeping position anyway because it will be too uncomfortable.

If you do shift onto your back, the discomfort will probably wake you up. Talk to your doctor, who may suggest that you use a pillow to keep yourself propped up on one side.

> Try experimenting with pillows to discover a comfortable sleeping position. Some women find that it helps to place a pillow under their abdomen or between their legs. Also, using a bunched-up pillow or rolled-up blanket at the small of your back may help to relieve some pressure. In fact, you'll see many "pregnancy pillows" on the market. If you're thinking about buying one, talk with your doctor first about which might work for you.

Tips For Sleeping Success

Although they might seem appealing when you're feeling desperate to get some ZZZs, remember that over-the-counter sleep aids, including herbal remedies, are not recommended for pregnant women.

Instead, these tips may safely improve your chances of getting a good night's sleep:

- Cut out caffeinated drinks like soda, coffee, and tea from your diet as much as possible. Restrict any intake of them to the morning or early afternoon.

- Avoid drinking a lot of fluids or eating a full meal within a few hours of going to bed. (But make sure that you also get plenty of nutrients and liquids throughout the day.) Some women find it helpful to eat more at breakfast and lunch and then have a smaller dinner. If nausea is keeping you up, try eating a few crackers before you go to bed.

- Get into a routine of going to bed and waking up at the same time each day.

- Avoid rigorous exercise right before you go to bed. Instead, do something relaxing, like reading a book or having a warm, caffeine-free drink, such as milk with honey or a cup of herbal tea.

- If a leg cramp awakens you, it may help to press your feet hard against the wall or to stand on the leg. Some women find that stretching their calf muscles before bed helps. Also, make sure that you're getting enough calcium and magnesium in your diet, which can help reduce leg cramps. But don't take any supplements without checking with your doctor.

- Take a yoga class or learn other relaxation techniques to help you unwind after a busy day. (Be sure to discuss any new activity or fitness regimen with your doctor first.)

- If fear and anxiety are keeping you awake, consider enrolling in a childbirth class or parenting class. More knowledge and the company of other pregnant women may help to ease the fears that are keeping you awake at night.

When You Can't Sleep

Of course, there are bound to be times when you just can't sleep. Instead of tossing and turning, worrying that you're not asleep, and counting the hours until your alarm clock will go off, get up and do something: read a book, listen to music, watch TV, catch up on letters or email, or pursue some other activity you enjoy. Eventually, you'll probably feel tired enough to get back to sleep.

And if possible, take short naps (30 to 60 minutes) during the day to make up for lost sleep. It won't be long before your baby will be setting the sleep rules in your house, so you might as well get used to sleeping in spurts!

Chapter 22

Depression During And After Pregnancy

What Is Depression?

Depression is more than just feeling "blue" or "down in the dumps" for a few days. It's a serious illness that involves the brain. With depression, sad, anxious, or "empty" feelings don't go away and interfere with day-to-day life and routines. These feelings can be mild to severe. The good news is that most people with depression get better with treatment.

How Common Is Depression During And After Pregnancy

Depression is a common problem during and after pregnancy. About 13 percent of pregnant women and new mothers have depression.

As many as 1 in 9 women experience depression before, during, or after pregnancy.

(Source: "Maternal Depression," Centers for Disease Control and Prevention (CDC).)

Approximately 4 percent of fathers experience depression in the first year after their child's birth. By a child's 12th birthday, about 1 out of 5 fathers will have experienced one or more episodes of depression. Younger fathers, those with a history of depression, and those experiencing difficulties affording items such as a home or car were most likely to experience depression.

(Source: "Depression Among Women," Centers for Disease Control and Prevention (CDC).)

About This Chapter: This chapter includes text excerpted from "Depression During And After Pregnancy Fact Sheet," Office on Women's Health (OWH), U.S. Department of Health and Human Services (HHS), February 12, 2016.

How Do I Know If I Have Depression?

When you are pregnant or after you have a baby, you may be depressed and not know it. Some normal changes during and after pregnancy can cause symptoms similar to those of depression. But if you have any of the following symptoms of depression for more than 2 weeks, call your doctor:

- Feeling restless or moody
- Feeling sad, hopeless, and overwhelmed
- Crying a lot
- Having no energy or motivation
- Eating too little or too much
- Sleeping too little or too much
- Having trouble focusing or making decisions
- Having memory problems
- Feeling worthless and guilty
- Losing interest or pleasure in activities you used to enjoy
- Withdrawing from friends and family
- Having headaches, aches and pains, or stomach problems that don't go away

Your doctor can figure out if your symptoms are caused by depression or something else.

What Causes Depression? What About Postpartum Depression?

There is no single cause. Rather, depression likely results from a combination of factors:

- Depression is a mental illness that tends to run in families. Women with a family history of depression are more likely to have depression.
- Changes in brain chemistry or structure are believed to play a big role in depression.
- Stressful life events, such as death of a loved one, caring for an aging family member, abuse, and poverty, can trigger depression.
- Hormonal factors unique to women may contribute to depression in some women. We know that hormones directly affect the brain chemistry that controls emotions

and mood. We also know that women are at greater risk of depression at certain times in their lives, such as puberty, during and after pregnancy, and during perimenopause. Some women also have depressive symptoms right before their period.

Depression after childbirth is called postpartum depression. Hormonal changes may trigger symptoms of postpartum depression. When you are pregnant, levels of the female hormones estrogen and progesterone increase greatly. In the first 24 hours after childbirth, hormone levels quickly return to normal. Researchers think the big change in hormone levels may lead to depression. This is much like the way smaller hormone changes can affect a woman's moods before she gets her period.

Levels of thyroid hormones may also drop after giving birth. The thyroid is a small gland in the neck that helps regulate how your body uses and stores energy from food. Low levels of thyroid hormones can cause symptoms of depression. A simple blood test can tell if this condition is causing your symptoms. If so, your doctor can prescribe thyroid medicine.

Other factors may play a role in postpartum depression. You may feel:

- Tired after delivery
- Tired from a lack of sleep or broken sleep
- Overwhelmed with a new baby
- Doubts about your ability to be a good mother
- Stress from changes in work and home routines
- An unrealistic need to be a perfect mom
- Loss of who you were before having the baby
- Less attractive
- A lack of free time

Are Some Women More At Risk For Depression During And After Pregnancy?

Certain factors may increase your risk of depression during and after pregnancy:

- A personal history of depression or another mental illness
- A family history of depression or another mental illness
- A lack of support from family and friends

- Anxiety or negative feelings about the pregnancy

- Problems with a previous pregnancy or birth

- Marriage or money problems

- Stressful life events

- Young age

- Substance abuse

Women who are depressed during pregnancy have a greater risk of depression after giving birth. The U.S. Preventive Services Task Force (USPSTF) recommends screening for depression during and after pregnancy, regardless of a woman's risk factors for depression.

What Is The Difference Between "Baby Blues," Postpartum Depression, And Postpartum Psychosis?

Many women have the baby blues in the days after childbirth. If you have the baby blues, you may:

- Have mood swings

- Feel sad, anxious, or overwhelmed

- Have crying spells

- Lose your appetite

- Have trouble sleeping

The baby blues most often go away within a few days or a week. The symptoms are not severe and do not need treatment.

The symptoms of postpartum depression last longer and are more severe. Postpartum depression can begin anytime within the first year after childbirth. If you have postpartum depression, you may have any of the symptoms of depression listed above. Symptoms may also include:

- Thoughts of hurting the baby

- Thoughts of hurting yourself

- Not having any interest in the baby

Postpartum depression needs to be treated by a doctor.

Postpartum psychosis is rare. It occurs in about 1 to 4 out of every 1,000 births. It usually begins in the first 2 weeks after childbirth. Women who have bipolar disorder or another mental health problem called schizoaffective disorder have a higher risk for postpartum psychosis. Symptoms may include:

- Seeing things that aren't there

- Feeling confused

- Having rapid mood swings

- Trying to hurt yourself or your baby

What Should I Do If I Have Symptoms Of Depression During Or After Pregnancy?

Call your doctor if:

- Your baby blues don't go away after 2 weeks

- Symptoms of depression get more and more intense

- Symptoms of depression begin any time after delivery, even many months later

- It is hard for you to perform tasks at work or at home

- You cannot care for yourself or your baby

- You have thoughts of harming yourself or your baby

Your doctor can ask you questions to test for depression. Your doctor can also refer you to a mental health professional who specializes in treating depression.

Some women don't tell anyone about their symptoms. They feel embarrassed, ashamed, or guilty about feeling depressed when they are supposed to be happy. They worry they will be viewed as unfit parents.

Any woman may become depressed during pregnancy or after having a baby. It doesn't mean you are a bad or "not together" mom. You and your baby don't have to suffer. There is help.

Here are some other helpful tips:

- Rest as much as you can. Sleep when the baby is sleeping.

- Don't try to do too much or try to be perfect.

- Ask your partner, family, and friends for help.

- Make time to go out, visit friends, or spend time alone with your partner.

- Discuss your feelings with your partner, family, and friends.

- Talk with other mothers so you can learn from their experiences.

- Join a support group. Ask your doctor about groups in your area.

- Don't make any major life changes during pregnancy or right after giving birth. Major changes can cause unneeded stress. Sometimes big changes can't be avoided. When that happens, try to arrange support and help in your new situation ahead of time.

How Is Depression Treated?

The two common types of treatment for depression are:

1. **Talk therapy.** This involves talking to a therapist, psychologist, or social worker to learn to change how depression makes you think, feel, and act.

2. **Medicine.** Your doctor can prescribe an antidepressant medicine. These medicines can help relieve symptoms of depression.

These treatment methods can be used alone or together. If you are depressed, your depression can affect your baby. Getting treatment is important for you and your baby. Talk with your doctor about the benefits and risks of taking medicine to treat depression when you are pregnant or breastfeeding.

Did You Know?

If you take medicine for depression, stopping your medicine when you become pregnant can cause your depression to come back. Do not stop any prescribed medicines without first talking to your doctor. Not using medicine that you need may be harmful to you or your baby.

What Can Happen If Depression Is Not Treated?

Untreated depression can hurt you and your baby. Some women with depression have a hard time caring for themselves during pregnancy. They may:

- Eat poorly

- Not gain enough weight

- Have trouble sleeping

- Miss prenatal visits

- Not follow medical instructions

- Use harmful substances, like tobacco, alcohol, or illegal drugs

Depression during pregnancy can raise the risk of:

- Problems during pregnancy or delivery

- Having a low-birth-weight baby

- Premature birth

Untreated postpartum depression can affect your ability to parent. You may:

- Lack energy

- Have trouble focusing

- Feel moody

- Not be able to meet your child's needs

As a result, you may feel guilty and lose confidence in yourself as a mother. These feelings can make your depression worse.

Researchers believe postpartum depression in a mother can affect her baby. It can cause the baby to have:

- Delays in language development

- Problems with mother-child bonding

- Behavior problems

- Increased crying

It helps if your partner or another caregiver can help meet the baby's needs while you are depressed.

All children deserve the chance to have a healthy mom. And all moms deserve the chance to enjoy their life and their children. If you are feeling depressed during pregnancy or after having a baby, don't suffer alone. Please tell a loved one and call your doctor right away.

Chapter 23
Medicines And Pregnancy

Is It Safe To Use Medicine While I Am Pregnant?

There is no clear-cut answer to this question. Before you start or stop any medicine, it is always best to speak with the doctor who is caring for you while you are pregnant. Read on to learn about deciding to use medicine while pregnant.

How Should I Decide Whether To Use A Medicine While I Am Pregnant?

When deciding whether or not to use a medicine in pregnancy, you and your doctor need to talk about the medicine's benefits and risks.

- **Benefits:** what are the good things the medicine can do for me and my growing baby (fetus)?

- **Risks:** what are the ways the medicine might harm me or my growing baby (fetus)?

There may be times during pregnancy when using medicine is a choice. Some of the medicine choices you and your doctor make while you are pregnant may differ from the choices you make when you are not pregnant. For example, if you get a cold, you may decide to "live with" your stuffy nose instead of using the "stuffy nose" medicine you use when you are not pregnant.

Other times, using medicine is not a choice—it is needed. Some women need to use medicines while they are pregnant. Sometimes, women need medicine for a few days or a couple

About This Chapter: This chapter includes text excerpted from "Pregnancy And Medicines Fact Sheet," Office on Women's Health (OWH), U.S. Department of Health and Human Services (HHS), July 16, 2012. Reviewed March 2017.

of weeks to treat a problem like a bladder infection or strep throat. Other women need to use medicine every day to control long-term health problems like asthma, diabetes, depression, or seizures. Also, some women have a pregnancy problem that needs treatment with medicine. These problems might include severe nausea and vomiting, earlier pregnancy losses, or preterm labor.

Where Do Doctors And Nurses Find Out About Using Medicines During Pregnancy?

Doctors and nurses get information from medicine labels and packages, textbooks, and research journals. They also share knowledge with other doctors and nurses and talk to the people who make and sell medicines.

The U.S. Food and Drug Administration (FDA) is the part of our country's government that controls the medicines that can and can't be sold in the United States. The FDA lets a company sell a medicine in the United States if it is safe to use and works for a certain health problem. Companies that make medicines usually have to show FDA doctors and scientists whether birth defects or other problems occur in baby animals when the medicine is given to pregnant animals. Most of the time, drugs are not studied in pregnant women.

The FDA works with the drug companies to make clear and complete medicine labels. But in most cases, there is not much information about how a medicine affects pregnant women and their growing babies. Many prescription medicine labels include the results of studies done in pregnant animals. But a medicine does not always affect growing humans and animals in the same way. Here is an example:

A medicine is given to pregnant rats. If the medicine causes problems in some of the rat babies, it may or may not cause problems in human babies. If there are no problems in the rat babies, it does not prove that the medicine will not cause problems in human babies.

The FDA asks for studies in two different kinds of animals. This improves the chance that the studies can predict what may happen in pregnant women and their babies.

There is a lot that FDA doctors and scientists do not know about using medicine during pregnancy. In a perfect world, every medicine label would include helpful information about the medicine's effects on pregnant women and their growing babies. Unfortunately, this is not the case.

How Do Prescription And Over-The-Counter (OTC) Medicine Labels Help My Doctor Choose The Right Medicine For Me When I Am Pregnant?

Doctors use information from many sources when they choose medicine for a patient, including medicine labels. To help doctors, the FDA created pregnancy letter categories to help explain what is known about using medicine during pregnancy. This system assigns letter categories to all prescription medicines. The letter category is listed in the label of a prescription medicine. The label states whether studies were done in pregnant women or pregnant animals and if so, what happened. Over-the-counter (OTC) medicines do not have a pregnancy letter category. Some OTC medicines were prescription medicines first and used to have a letter category. Talk to your doctor and follow the instructions on the label before taking OTC medicines.

Prescription Medicines

The FDA chooses a medicine's letter category based on what is known about the medicine when used in pregnant women and animals.

Table 23.1. Definition Of Medicine Categories

Pregnancy Category	Definition	Examples Of Drugs
A	In human studies, pregnant women used the medicine and their babies did not have any problems related to using the medicine.	• Folic acid • Levothyroxine (thyroid hormone medicine)
B	In humans, there are no good studies. But in animal studies, pregnant animals received the medicine, and the babies did not show any problems related to the medicine. **Or** In animal studies, pregnant animals received the medicine, and some babies had problems. But in human studies, pregnant women used the medicine and their babies did not have any problems related to using the medicine.	• Some antibiotics like amoxicillin. • Zofran (ondansetron) for nausea • Glucophage (metformin) for diabetes • Some insulins used to treat diabetes such as regular and NPH insulin.

Table 23.1. Continued

Pregnancy Category	Definition	Examples Of Drugs
C	In humans, there are no good studies. In animals, pregnant animals treated with the medicine had some babies with problems. However, sometimes the medicine may still help the human mothers and babies more than it might harm. **Or** No animal studies have been done, and there are no good studies in pregnant women.	• Diflucan (fluconazole) for yeast infections • Ventolin (albuterol) for asthma • Zoloft (sertraline) and • Prozac (fluoxetine) for depression
D	Studies in humans and other reports show that when pregnant women use the medicine, some babies are born with problems related to the medicine. However, in some serious situations, the medicine may still help the mother and the baby more than it might harm.	• Paxil (paroxetine) for depression • Lithium for bipolar disorder • Dilantin (phenytoin) for epileptic seizures • Some cancer chemotherapy
X	Studies or reports in humans or animals show that mothers using the medicine during pregnancy may have babies with problems related to the medicine. There are no situations where the medicine can help the mother or baby enough to make the risk of problems worth it. These medicines should never be used by pregnant women.	• Accutane (isotretinoin) for cystic acne • Thalomid (thalidomide) for a type of skin disease

The FDA is working hard to gather more knowledge about using medicine during pregnancy. The FDA is also trying to make medicine labels more helpful to doctors. Medicine label information for prescription medicines is now changing, and the pregnancy part of the label will change over the next few years. As this prescription information is updated, it is added to an online information clearinghouse called DailyMed that gives up-to-date, free information to consumers and healthcare providers.

OTC Medicines

All OTC medicines have a drug facts label. The Drug Facts label is arranged the same way on all OTC medicines. This makes information about using the medicine easier to find. One section of the Drug Facts label is for pregnant women. With OTC medicines, the label usually tells a pregnant woman to speak with her doctor before using the medicine. Some OTC medicines are known to cause certain problems in pregnancy. The labels for these medicines give pregnant women facts about why and when they should not use the medicine. Here are some examples:

- Nonsteroidal anti-inflammatory drugs (NSAIDs) like ibuprofen (Advil, Motrin), naproxen (Aleve), and aspirin (acetylsalicylate), can cause serious blood flow problems in the baby if used during the last 3 months of pregnancy (after 28 weeks). Also, aspirin may increase the chance for bleeding problems in the mother and the baby during pregnancy or at delivery.

- The labels for nicotine therapy drugs, like the nicotine patch and lozenge, remind women that smoking can harm an unborn child. While the medicine is thought to be safer than smoking, the risks of the medicine are not fully known. Pregnant smokers are told to try quitting without the medicine first.

> Things like caffeine, vitamins, and herbal remedies can affect the growing fetus. Talk with your doctor about cutting down on caffeine and ask which type of vitamin you should take. Never use an herbal product without talking to your doctor first.

What If I'm Thinking About Getting Pregnant?

If you are not pregnant yet, you can help your chances for having a healthy baby by planning ahead. Schedule a pre-pregnancy checkup. At this visit, you can talk to your doctor about the medicines, vitamins, and herbs you use. It is very important that you keep treating your health problems while you are pregnant. Your doctor can tell you if you need to switch your medicine. Ask about vitamins for women who are trying to get pregnant. All women who can get pregnant should take a daily vitamin with folic acid (a B vitamin) to prevent birth defects of the brain and spinal cord. You should begin taking these vitamins before you become pregnant or if you could become pregnant. It is also a good idea to discuss caffeine, alcohol, and smoking with your doctor at this time.

Is It Safe To Use Medicine While I Am Trying To Become Pregnant?

It is hard to know exactly when you will get pregnant. Once you do get pregnant, you may not know you are pregnant for 10 to 14 days or longer. Before you start trying to get pregnant, it is wise to schedule a meeting with your doctor to discuss medicines that you use daily or every now and then. Sometimes, medicines should be changed, and sometimes they can be stopped before a woman gets pregnant. Each woman is different. So you should discuss your medicines with your doctor rather than making medicine changes on your own.

- Do not stop any prescribed medicines without first talking to your doctor.
- Talk to your doctor before using any over-the-counter medicine.

What If I Get Sick And Need To Use Medicine While I Am Pregnant?

Whether or not you should use medicine during pregnancy is a serious question to discuss with your doctor. Some health problems need treatment. Not using a medicine that you need could harm you and your baby. For example, a urinary tract infection (UTI) that is not treated may become a kidney infection. Kidney infections can cause preterm labor and low birth weight. You need an antibiotic to cure a UTI. Ask your doctor whether the benefits of taking a certain medicine outweigh the risks for you and your baby.

I Have A Health Problem. Should I Stop Using My Medicine While I Am Pregnant?

If you are pregnant or thinking about becoming pregnant, you should talk to your doctor about your medicines. Do not stop or change them on your own. This includes medicines for depression, asthma, diabetes, seizures (epilepsy), and other health problems. Not using medicine that you need may be more harmful to you and your baby than using the medicine.

For women living with human immunodeficiency virus (HIV), the Centers for Disease Control and Prevention (CDC) recommends using *zidovudine* (AZT) during pregnancy. Studies show that HIV positive women who use AZT during pregnancy greatly lower the risk of passing HIV to their babies. If a diabetic woman does not use her medicine during pregnancy, she raises her risk for miscarriage, stillbirth, and some birth defects. If asthma and high blood pressure are not controlled during pregnancy, problems with the fetus may result.

Are Vitamins Safe For Me While I Am Pregnant?

Women who are pregnant should not take regular vitamins. They can contain doses that are too high. Ask about special vitamins for pregnant women that can help keep you and your baby healthy. These prenatal vitamins should contain at least 400–800 micrograms (μg) of folic acid. It is best to start taking these vitamins before you become pregnant or if you could become pregnant. Folic acid reduces the chance of a baby having a neural tube defect, like spina bifida, where the spine or brain does not form the right way. It's important to take the vitamin dose prescribed by your doctor. Too many vitamins can harm your baby. For example, very high levels of vitamin A have been linked with severe birth defects.

Are Herbs, Minerals, Or Amino Acids Safe For Me While I Am Pregnant?

No one is sure if these are safe for pregnant women, so it's best not to use them. Even some "natural" products may not be good for women who are pregnant or breastfeeding. Except for some vitamins, little is known about using dietary supplements while pregnant. Some herbal remedy labels claim that they will help with pregnancy. But, most often there are no good studies to show if these claims are true or if the herb can cause harm to you or your baby. Talk with your doctor before using any herbal product or dietary supplement. These products may contain things that could harm you or your growing baby during your pregnancy.

In the United States, there are different laws for medicines and for dietary supplements. The part of the FDA that controls dietary supplements is the same part that controls foods sold in the United States. Only dietary supplements containing new dietary ingredients that were not marketed before October 15, 1994 submit safety information for review by the FDA. However, unlike medicines, the FDA does not approve herbal remedies and "natural products" for safety or for what they say they will do. Most have not even been evaluated for their potential to cause harm to you or the growing fetus, let alone shown to be safe for use in pregnancy. Before a company can sell a medicine, the company must complete many studies and send the results to the FDA. Many scientists and doctors at the FDA check the study results. The FDA allows the medicine to be sold only if the studies show that the medicine works and is safe to use.

Chapter 24
X-Rays During Pregnancy

Pregnancy is a time to take good care of yourself and your unborn child. Many things are especially important during pregnancy, such as eating right, cutting out cigarettes and alcohol, and being careful about the prescription and over-the-counter drugs you take. Diagnostic X-rays and other medical radiation procedures of the *abdominal area* also deserve extra attention during pregnancy.

Diagnostic X-rays can give the doctor important and even life-saving information about a person's medical condition. But like many things, diagnostic X-rays have risks as well as benefits. They should be used only when they will give the doctor information needed to treat you.

You'll probably never need an abdominal X-ray during pregnancy. But sometimes, because of a particular medical condition, your physician may feel that a diagnostic X-ray of your abdomen or lower torso is needed. If this should happen—don't be upset. The risk to you and your unborn child is very small, and the benefit of finding out about your medical condition is far greater. In fact, the risk of not having a needed X-ray could be much greater than the risk from the radiation. But even small risks should not be taken if they're unnecessary.

You can reduce those risks by telling your doctor if you are, or think you might be, pregnant whenever an abdominal X-ray is prescribed. If you are pregnant, the doctor may decide that it would be best to cancel the X-ray examination, to postpone it, or to modify it to reduce the amount of radiation. Or, depending on your medical needs, and realizing that the risk is very small, the doctor may feel that it is best to proceed with the X-ray as planned. In any case, you should feel free to discuss the decision with your doctor.

About This Chapter: This chapter includes text excerpted from "X-Rays, Pregnancy And You," U.S. Food and Drug Administration (FDA), February 9, 2016.

What Kind Of X-Rays Can Affect The Unborn Child?

During most X-ray examinations—like those of the arms, legs, head, teeth, or chest—your reproductive organs are not exposed to the direct X-ray beam. So these kinds of procedures, when properly done, do not involve any risk to the unborn child. However, X-rays of the mother's lower torso—abdomen, stomach, pelvis, lower back, or kidneys—may expose the unborn child to the direct X-ray beam. They are of more concern.

What Are The Possible Effects Of X-Rays?

There is scientific disagreement about whether the small amounts of radiation used in diagnostic radiology can actually harm the unborn child, but it is known that the unborn child is very sensitive to the effects of things like radiation, certain drugs, excess alcohol, and infection. This is true, in part, because the cells are rapidly dividing and growing into specialized cells and tissues. If radiation or other agents were to cause changes in these cells, there could be a slightly increased chance of birth defects or certain illnesses, such as leukemia, later in life.

It should be pointed out, however, that the majority of birth defects and childhood diseases occur even if the mother is not exposed to any known harmful agent during pregnancy. Scientists believe that heredity and random errors in the developmental process are responsible for most of these problems.

What If I'm X-Rayed Before I Know I'm Pregnant?

Don't be alarmed. Remember that the possibility of any harm to you and your unborn child from an X-ray is very small. There are, however, rare situations in which a woman who is unaware of her pregnancy may receive a very large number of abdominal X-rays over a short period. Or she may receive radiation treatment of the lower torso. Under these circumstances, the woman should discuss the possible risks with her doctor.

How You Can Help Minimize The Risks

- **Most important, tell your physician if you are pregnant or think you might be.** This is important for many medical decisions, such as drug prescriptions and nuclear medicine procedures, as well as X-rays. And remember, this is true even in the very early weeks of pregnancy.

- Occasionally, a woman may mistake the symptoms of pregnancy for the symptoms of a disease. If you have any of the symptoms of pregnancy—nausea, vomiting, breast tenderness, fatigue—consider whether you might be pregnant and tell your doctor or X-ray technologist (the person doing the examination) before having an X-ray of the lower torso. A pregnancy test may be called for.

- If you are pregnant, or think you might be, do not hold a child who is being X-rayed. If you are not pregnant and you are asked to hold a child during an X-ray, be sure to ask for a lead apron to protect your reproductive organs. This is to prevent damage to your genes that could be passed on and cause harmful effects in your future descendants.

- Whenever an X-ray is requested, tell your doctor about any similar X-rays you have had recently. It may not be necessary to do another. It is a good idea to keep a record of the X-ray examinations you and your family have had taken so you can provide this kind of information accurately.

- Feel free to talk with your doctor about the need for an X-ray examination. You should understand the reason X-rays are requested in your particular case.

Chapter 25

Food Poisoning During Pregnancy

Food Safety For Pregnant Women

When pregnant, a woman's immune system is reduced. This places her and her unborn baby at increased risk of contracting the bacteria, viruses, and parasites that cause foodborne illness. Foodborne illnesses can be worse during pregnancy and may lead to miscarriage or premature delivery. Maternal foodborne illness can also lead to death or severe health problems in newborn babies. Some foodborne illnesses, such as *Listeria* and *Toxoplasma gondii*, can infect the fetus even if the mother does not feel sick. This is why doctors provide pregnant women with specific guidelines to foods that they should and should not eat.

Table 25.1. Foodborne Pathogen And Illness's Impact During Pregnancy

Foodborne Pathogen	Foodborne Illness's Impact During Pregnancy
Campylobacter	• Infections usually result in severe diarrhea and in pregnant women the infection usually are mild and have no adverse consequences for mother or child.
	• Infection during the third trimester has a higher chance of leading to neonatal sepsis because the bacterium is able to transmit to the baby during time of delivery.
	• In some cases, infection in the early stages of pregnancy can cause miscarriages and premature birth.
E. coli	• The main concern of *E. coli* infection during pregnancy is dehydration though in rare cases severe complications may arise.

About This Chapter: This chapter includes text excerpted from "Food Safety For Pregnant Women," Foodsafety. gov, U.S. Department of Health and Human Services (HHS), June 4, 2015.

Table 25.1. Continued

Foodborne Pathogen	Foodborne Illness's Impact During Pregnancy
Listeria	• *Listeria* can cause Listeriosis, an infection that may cause miscarriages, premature labor, the delivery of low-birth-weight infants, or infant death.
	• The infection can pass to a fetus even if the mother does not show signs of infection.
	• Pregnant women are about 10 times more likely than the general population to get a *Listeria* infection.
	• A fetus infected with *Listeria* may develop health problems later in life including:
	• intellectual disability,
	• paralysis,
	• seizures,
	• blindness,
	• or impairments of brain, heart, or kidney.
Salmonella	• Infection can lead to health complications during pregnancy, including dehydration and bacteremia (bacteria in the blood) which can lead to meningitis.
	• *Salmonella* can pass to the baby during pregnancy. Babies born with *Salmonella* infection may have diarrhea and fever after birth and may develop more serve complications meningitis.
Toxoplasma gondii (toxoplasmosis)	• If infection occurs during pregnancy, babies can develop:
	• hearing loss,
	• intellectual disability,
	• and blindness.
	• Some children can develop brain or eye problems years after birth.
	• The infection can pass to a fetus even if the mother does not show signs of infection.

What You Can Do During Pregnancy

Choose Your Seafood Carefully

Fish and other seafood are excellent sources of protein and omega-3 fatty acids that are important for fetus development. According to the U.S. Food and Drug Administration (FDA), the high quality of protein, many minerals, omega-3 fatty acids, combined with mostly low levels

Symptoms Of Foodborne Illness

Symptoms vary, but may include stomach pain, vomiting, and/or diarrhea. Sometimes foodborne illness is confused with the flu because the symptoms can be flu like with a fever, headache, and body aches.

(Source: "While You're Pregnant—What Is Foodborne Illness?" U.S. Food and Drug Administration (FDA).)

of saturated fat found in fish can play an important role in the growth and development of a baby before birth. It is important for proper development to consume fish, but pregnant women should still avoid fish heavy in methylmercury. High levels of methylmercury act as a neurotoxin that can be harmful to the nervous system. A fetus's developing nervous system is particularly vulnerable.

The following fish potentially contain high levels of mercury that could harm the development of her baby's nervous system and should be avoided:

- Swordfish

- Shark

- King Mackerel

- Tilefish (golden tilefish)

It is important for fetal development to avoid fish high in mercury, but pregnant women should not avoid fish altogether. According to the 2010 Dietary Guidelines for Americans, a pregnant woman should try to consume up to 12 ounces a week of fish and shellfish that are lower in mercury. Seafood lower in mercury includes:

- Shrimp

- Salmon

- Pollock

- Catfish

- Canned light tuna

- Pangasius

- Tilapia

- Cod

- Clams

- Crab

> While pregnant women can consume albacore tuna and tuna steaks, they should limit their tuna intake to 6 ounces a week. This is because some testing has shown that tuna can have high mercury levels that could lead to poor fetal development.

Avoid Raw Seafood

Raw seafood may contain parasites or bacteria including *Listeria* that can make a pregnant woman ill and could potentially harm her baby. All seafood dishes should be cooked to 145°F. This means that she should avoid:

- Sushi

- Sashimi

- Raw Oysters

- Raw Clams

- Raw Scallops

- Ceviche

Be Selective With Smoked Seafood

Refrigerated smoked seafood presents a very real threat of *Listeria*. Refrigerated smoked seafood, such as salmon, trout, whitefish, cod, tuna, or mackerel are often labeled as:

- Nova-style

- Lox

- Kippered

- Smoked, or

- Jerky

Refrigerated smoked fish should be reheated to 165°F before eating.

It is okay to eat smoked seafood during pregnancy if it is canned, shelf stable or an ingredient in a casserole or other cooked dish.

Avoid Unpasteurized Juice Or Cider

Unpasteurized juice, even fresh squeezed juice, and cider can cause foodborne illness. In particular these beverages have been linked to outbreaks of *E. coli*. In addition, *E. coli 0157:H7* infections have been associated with unpasteurized juice. This strain of *E. coli* can result in liver failure and death. Individuals with reduced immunity are particularly susceptible. To prevent *E. coli* infection, either choose a pasteurized version or bring unpasteurized juice or cider to a rolling boil and boil for at least 1 minute before drinking.

Unpasteurized Milk Is A No-No

Milk that has not been pasteurized may contain bacteria such as *Campylobacter, E. coli, Listeria, Salmonella* or tuberculosis. To avoid getting these foodborne illnesses, drink only pasteurized milk.

Avoid Soft Cheese And Cheese Made From Unpasteurized Milk

Soft cheeses in particular tend to be made with unpasteurized milk. When pregnant, a woman should avoid the following cheeses that tend to be made with unpasteurized milk:

- Brie
- Feta
- Camembert
- Roquefort
- Queso Blanco, and
- Queso fresco

Cheese made with unpasteurized milk may contain *E. coli* or *Listeria*. Instead of eating soft cheese, eat hard cheese such as Cheddar or Swiss. If a pregnant woman wants to continue to eat soft cheese, she should make sure to check the label to ensure that the cheese is made from pasteurized milk. Pregnant woman should pay particular attention at farmers markets to make sure that fresh and soft cheeses are pasteurized.

Only Consume Cooked Eggs

Undercooked eggs may contain *Salmonella*. To safely consume eggs, cook them until the yolks are firm that way you know *Salmonella* has been destroyed. If you are making a casserole or other dish containing eggs, make sure the dish is cooked to a temperature of 160°F. Foods that may contain raw eggs should be avoided. They are as follows:

- Eggnog
- Raw batter
- Caesar salad dressing
- Tiramisu
- Eggs Benedict
- Homemade ice cream
- Freshly made or homemade hollandaise sauce

Any batter that contains raw eggs, such as cookie, cake or brownie batter, should not be consumed uncooked by pregnant women. The batter may contain *Salmonella* which can make a pregnant woman very sick. To safely consume these yummy treats, bake them thoroughly. No matter how tempting, DO NOT lick the spoon.

Avoid Premade Meat Or Seafood Salad

When pregnant, a woman should not purchase premade ham salad, chicken salad, or seafood salad which may contain *Listeria*. These items are commonly found in delis. She can safely consume these yummy lunch items by making the salads at home and following the food safety basics of clean, separate, cook and chill.

Tailor Your Homemade Ice Cream Recipe

Homemade ice cream may contain uncooked eggs, which may contain *Salmonella*. To make homemade ice cream safer, use pasteurized shell eggs, a pasteurized egg product or a recipe with a cooked custard base.

Do Not Eat Raw Sprouts

Raw or undercooked sprouts, such as alfalfa, clover, mung bean, and radish may contain *E. coli* or *Salmonella*. If a pregnant woman would like to eat sprouts safely, she should cook them thoroughly.

Avoid Undercooked Meat And Poultry

All meat and poultry should be thoroughly cooked before eating. A food thermometer should be used to ensure that the meat has reached the U.S. Department of Agriculture (USDA) recommended safe minimum internal temperature.

Table 25.2. Minimum Cooking Temperatures

Category	Food	Temperature (°F)	Rest Time*
Ground Meat and Meat Mixtures	Beef, Pork, Veal, Lamb	160	None
	Turkey, Chicken	165	None
Fresh Beef, Veal, Lamb	Steaks, roasts, chops	145	3 minutes
Poultry	Chicken & Turkey, whole	165	None
	Poultry breasts, roasts	165	None
	Poultry thighs, legs, wings	165	None
	Duck & Goose	165	None
	Stuffing (cooked alone or in bird)	165	None
Pork and Ham	Fresh pork	145	3 minutes
	Fresh ham (raw)	145	3 minutes
	Precooked ham (to reheat)	140	None
Eggs and Egg Dishes	Eggs	Cook until yolk and white are firm	None
	Egg dishes	160	None
Leftovers and Casseroles	Leftovers	165	None
	Casseroles	165	None
Seafood	Fin Fish	145 or cook until flesh is opaque and separates easily with a fork.	None
	Shrimp, lobster, and crabs	Cook until flesh is pearly and opaque.	None
	Clams, oysters, and mussels	Cook until shells open during cooking.	None
	Scallops	Cook until flesh is milky white or opaque and firm.	None

* *After you remove meat from a grill, oven, or other heat source, allow it to rest for the specified amount of time. During the rest time, its temperature remains constant or continues to rise, which destroys harmful germs.*

Following the minimum recommended internal temperature is important because meat and poultry may contain *E. coli, Salmonella, Campylobacter, Toxoplasma gondii.*

According to the Centers for Disease Control and Prevention (CDC), 50 percent of toxoplasmosis cases are believed to be caused by eating contaminated meat. The CDC recommends the following preventive measures to reduce the risk of contracting toxoplasmosis from meat consumption:

- Cook meat to the USDA recommended minimum safe internal temperature.

- Freeze meat for several days at sub-zero (0°F) temperatures before cooking to greatly reduce chance of infection.

- Wash cutting boards, dishes, counters, utensils, and hands with hot soapy water after contact with raw meat, poultry, seafood, or unwashed fruits or vegetables.

Reheat Hot Dogs And Luncheon Meats

While the label may say precooked on the following products, a pregnant woman should reheat these meats to steaming hot or 165°F before eating. These meat items may contain *Listeria* and are unsafe to eat if they have not been thoroughly reheated.

- Hot dogs

- Luncheon meats

- Cold cuts

- Fermented or dry sausage

- Any other deli-style meat and poultry

Be Selective With Meat Spreads Or Pate

Unpasteurized meat spreads or pate may contain *Listeria*. To consume these products safely when pregnant, eat canned versions. Do not eat refrigerated pates or meat spreads as they have a high likelihood of containing *Listeria*.

Four Basic Steps To Food Safety

1. Clean: Wash hands and surfaces often
2. Separate: Don't cross-contaminate
3. Cook: Cook to safe temperatures
4. Chill: Refrigerate promptly

(Source: "Food Safety For Pregnant Women," U.S. Food and Drug Administration (FDA).)

Chapter 26
Drinking Alcohol During Pregnancy

Alcohol Use In Pregnancy

There is no known safe amount of alcohol use during pregnancy or while trying to get pregnant. There is also no safe time during pregnancy to drink. All types of alcohol are equally harmful, including all wines and beer. When a pregnant woman drinks alcohol, so does her baby.

Women also should not drink alcohol if they are sexually active and do not use effective contraception (birth control). This is because a woman might get pregnant and expose her baby to alcohol before she knows she is pregnant. Nearly half of all pregnancies in the United States are unplanned. Most women will not know they are pregnant for up to 4 to 6 weeks.

Fetal alcohol spectrum disorders (FASDs) are completely preventable if a woman does not drink alcohol during pregnancy. Why take the risk?

Why Alcohol Is Dangerous

Alcohol in the mother's blood passes to the baby through the umbilical cord. Drinking alcohol during pregnancy can cause miscarriage, stillbirth, and a range of lifelong physical, behavioral, and intellectual disabilities. These disabilities are known as fetal alcohol spectrum disorders (FASDs). Children with FASDs might have the following characteristics and behaviors:

- Abnormal facial features, such as a smooth ridge between the nose and upper lip (this ridge is called the philtrum)

About This Chapter: Text beginning with the heading "Alcohol Use In Pregnancy" is excerpted from "Alcohol Use In Pregnancy," Centers for Disease Control and Prevention (CDC), July 21, 2016; Text under the heading "Frequently Asked Questions" is excerpted from "Alcohol And Pregnancy Questions And Answers," Centers for Disease Control and Prevention (CDC), October 24, 2016.

- Difficulty in school (especially with math)

- Difficulty with attention

- Hyperactive behavior

- Intellectual disability or low IQ

- Learning disabilities

- Low body weight

- Poor coordination

- Poor memory

- Poor reasoning and judgment skills

- Problems with the heart, kidney, or bones

- Shorter-than-average height

- Sleep and sucking problems as a baby

- Small head size

- Speech and language delays

- Vision or hearing problems

> FASDs are not genetic or hereditary. If a woman drinks alcohol during her pregnancy, her baby can be born with an FASD. But if a woman has an FASD, her own child cannot have an FASD, unless she drinks alcohol during pregnancy.
>
> _(Source: "Alcohol And Pregnancy Questions And Answers," Centers for Disease Control and Prevention (CDC).)_

When Alcohol Is Dangerous

There is no safe time to drink alcohol during pregnancy. Alcohol can cause problems for the developing baby throughout pregnancy, including before a woman knows she is pregnant. Drinking alcohol in the first three months of pregnancy can cause the baby to have abnormal facial features. Growth and central nervous system problems (e.g., low birthweight, behavioral problems) can occur from drinking alcohol anytime during pregnancy. The baby's brain is developing throughout pregnancy and can be affected by exposure to alcohol at any time.

If a woman is drinking alcohol during pregnancy, it is never too late to stop. The sooner a woman stops drinking, the better it will be for both her baby and herself.

Frequently Asked Questions

I Just Found Out I Am Pregnant. I Have Stopped Drinking Now, But I Was Drinking In The First Few Weeks Of My Pregnancy, Before I Knew I Was Pregnant. What Should I Do Now?

The most important thing is that you have completely stopped drinking after learning of your pregnancy. It is never too late to stop drinking. Because brain growth takes place throughout pregnancy, the sooner you stop drinking the safer it will be for you and your baby.

If you drank any amount of alcohol while you were pregnant, talk with your child's healthcare provider as soon as possible and share your concerns. Make sure you get regular prenatal checkups.

What Is A "Drink"? What If I Drink Only Beer Or Wine Coolers?

Drinking any type of alcohol can affect your baby's growth and development and cause FASDs. This includes all wines, beer, and mixed drinks. A standard drink is defined as .60 ounces of pure alcohol. This is equivalent to one 12-ounce beer or wine cooler, one 5-ounce glass of wine, or 1.5 ounces of 80 proof distilled spirits (hard liquor). Some drinks, like mixed alcoholic drinks or malt liquor drinks, might have more alcohol in them than a 12-ounce beer.

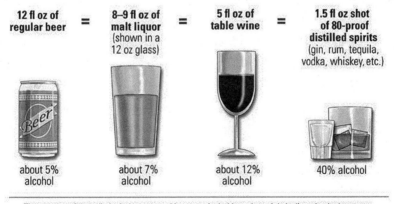

The percent of "pure" alcohol, expressed here as alcohol by volume (alc/vol), varies by beverage.

Figure 26.1. Standard Drink

(Source: "What Is A Standard Drink?" National Institute on Alcohol Abuse and Alcoholism (NIAAA).)

There is no safe kind of alcohol. If you have any questions about your alcohol use and its risks to your health, talk to your healthcare provider.

Is It Okay To Drink A Little Or At Certain Times During Pregnancy?

There is no known safe amount of alcohol use during your pregnancy or when you are trying to get pregnant. There is also no safe time to drink when you are pregnant. Alcohol can cause problems for your developing baby throughout your pregnancy, including before you know you are pregnant.

FASDs are completely preventable if a woman does not drink alcohol during pregnancy—so why take the risk?

I Drank Wine During My Last Pregnancy And My Baby Turned Out Fine. Why Shouldn't I Drink Again During This Pregnancy?

Every pregnancy is different. Drinking alcohol might affect one baby more than another. You could have one child who is born healthy and another child who is born with problems.

If I Drank When I Was Pregnant, Does That Mean My Baby Will Have An FASD?

If you drank any amount of alcohol while you were pregnant, talk with your child's healthcare provider as soon as possible and share your concerns.

You may not know right away if your child has been affected. FASDs include a range of physical and intellectual disabilities that are not always easy to identify when a child is a newborn. Some of these effects may not be known until your child is in school.

There is no cure for FASDs. However, identifying and intervening with children with these conditions as early as possible can help them to reach their full potential.

Is It Okay To Drink Alcohol If I Am Trying To Get Pregnant?

You might be pregnant and not know it yet. You probably won't know you are pregnant for up to 4 to 6 weeks. This means you might be drinking and exposing your baby to alcohol without meaning to. Alcohol use during pregnancy can also lead to miscarriage and stillbirth.

The best advice is to stop drinking alcohol when you start trying to get pregnant.

Why Should I Worry About Alcohol Use If I Am Not Pregnant And Not Trying To Get Pregnant?

If you drink alcohol and do not use contraception (birth control) when you have sex, you might get pregnant and expose your baby to alcohol before you know you are pregnant.

Nearly half of all pregnancies in the United States are unplanned. And many women do not know they are pregnant right away. So, if you are not trying to get pregnant but you are having sex, talk to your healthcare provider about using contraception consistently.

Can A Father's Drinking Cause Harm To The Baby?

How alcohol affects the male sperm is currently being studied. Whatever the effects are found to be, they are not fetal alcohol spectrum disorders (FASDs). FASDs are caused specifically by the mother's alcohol use during pregnancy.

However, the father's role is important. He can help the woman avoid drinking alcohol during pregnancy. He can encourage her to abstain from alcohol by avoiding social situations that involve drinking. He can also help her by avoiding alcohol himself.

I've Tried To Stop Drinking Before, But I Just Couldn't Do It. Where Can I Get Help?

If you cannot stop drinking, contact your doctor, local Alcoholics Anonymous (A.A.), or local alcohol treatment center.

Behavioral Health Treatment Services Locator

The Substance Abuse and Mental Health Services Administration (SAMHSA) has a treatment facility locator (findtreatment.samhsa.gov). This locator helps people find drug and alcohol treatment programs in their area.

Alcoholics Anonymous (A.A.)

Alcoholics Anonymous® is a fellowship of men and women who share their experience, strength and hope with each other that they may solve their common problem and help others to recover from alcoholism.

I Suspect My Child Might Have An FASD. What Should I Do?

If you think your child might have an FASD, talk to your child's doctor and share your concerns. Don't wait!

If you or the doctor thinks there could be a problem, ask the doctor for a referral to a specialist (someone who knows about FASDs), such as a developmental pediatrician, child psychologist, or clinical geneticist. In some cities, there are clinics whose staffs have special training in diagnosing and treating children with FASDs. To find doctors and clinics in your area visit the National and State Resource Directory (www.nofas.org/resource-directory) from the National Organization on Fetal Alcohol Syndrome (NOFAS).

At the same time as you ask the doctor for a referral to a specialist, **call your state's public early childhood system** to request a free evaluation to find out if your child qualifies for intervention services. This is sometimes called a *Child Find* evaluation. You do not need to wait for a doctor's referral or a medical diagnosis to make this call.

Where to call for a free evaluation from the state depends on your child's age:

- **If your child is younger than 3 years old,** contact your local early intervention system (www.cdc.gov/ncbddd/actearly/parents/states.html).

- **If your child is 3 years old or older,** contact your local public school system.

Even if your child is not old enough for kindergarten or enrolled in a public school, call your local elementary school or board of education and ask to speak with someone who can help you have your child evaluated.

Chapter 27

Smoking During Pregnancy

How Does Smoking During Pregnancy Harm My Health And My Baby?

Most people know that smoking causes cancer, heart disease, and other major health problems. Smoking during pregnancy causes additional health problems, including premature birth (being born too early), certain birth defects, and infant death.

Smoking Statistics

Women in their early 20s (aged 20–24) had the highest smoking rate before pregnancy (16.8%) of all age groups, followed by teenagers (13.5%).

(Source: "Smoking Prevalence And Cessation Before And During Pregnancy: Data From The Birth Certificate, 2014," National Vital Statistics Reports (NVSR), Centers for Disease Control and Prevention (CDC).)

- Smoking makes it harder for a woman to get pregnant.

- Women who smoke during pregnancy are more likely than other women to have a miscarriage.

- Smoking can cause problems with the placenta—the source of the baby's food and oxygen during pregnancy. For example, the placenta can separate from the womb too early, causing bleeding, which is dangerous to the mother and baby.

About This Chapter: This chapter includes text excerpted from "Tobacco Use And Pregnancy," Centers for Disease Control and Prevention (CDC), July 20, 2016.

- Smoking during pregnancy can cause a baby to be born too early or to have low birth weight—making it more likely the baby will be sick and have to stay in the hospital longer. A few babies may even die.

- Smoking during and after pregnancy is a risk factor of Sudden Infant Death Syndrome (SIDS). SIDS is an infant death for which a cause of the death cannot be found.

- Babies born to women who smoke are more likely to have certain birth defects, like a cleft lip or cleft palate.

What Are E-Cigarettes? Are They Safer Than Regular Cigarettes In Pregnancy?

Electronic cigarettes (also called electronic nicotine delivery systems or e-cigarettes) come in different sizes and shapes, including "pens," "mods," (i.e., these types are modified by the user) and "tanks." Most e-cigarettes contain a battery, a heating device, and a cartridge to hold liquid. The liquid typically contains nicotine, flavorings, and other chemicals. The battery-powered device heats the liquid in the cartridge into an aerosol that the user inhales.

Although the aerosol of e-cigarettes generally has fewer harmful substances than cigarette smoke, e-cigarettes and other products containing nicotine are not safe to use during pregnancy. Nicotine is a health danger for pregnant women and developing babies and can damage a developing baby's brain and lungs. Also, some of the flavorings used in e-cigarettes may be harmful to a developing baby.

What Are The Benefits Of Quitting?

Quitting smoking will help you feel better and provide a healthier environment for your baby.

When you stop smoking

- Your baby will get more oxygen, even after just one day of not smoking.

- There is less risk that your baby will be born too early.

- There is a better chance that your baby will come home from the hospital with you.

- You will be less likely to develop heart disease, stroke, lung cancer, chronic lung disease, and other smoke-related diseases.

- You will be more likely to live to know your grandchildren.

- You will have more energy and breathe more easily.

- Your clothes, hair, and home will smell better.

- Your food will taste better.

- You will have more money that you can spend on other things.

- You will feel good about what you have done for yourself and your baby.

Quitting Smoking Can Be Hard, But It Is One Of The Best Ways A Woman Can Protect Herself And Her Baby's Health

If you or someone you know wants to quit smoking, talk to your doctor, nurse, or health-care provider about strategies. For support in quitting, including free quit coaching, a free quit plan, free educational materials, and referrals to local resources, please call 800-QUIT-NOW (800-784-8669).

Smoking Cessation Statistics

- Although teenagers had the second-highest prepregnancy smoking rate (13.5%) by maternal age group after women aged 20–24 (16.8%), they had the highest smoking cessation rate of all age groups at 26.4 percent.

- Similar to the findings for smoking cessation before pregnancy, teenagers had the second-highest smoking rate during pregnancy by maternal age group (10.1%) after women aged 20–24 (13.0%), but the highest rate of smoking cessation during pregnancy (27.2%).

(Source: "Smoking Prevalence And Cessation Before And During Pregnancy: Data From The Birth Certificate, 2014," National Vital Statistics Reports (NVSR), Centers for Disease Control and Prevention (CDC).)

How Does Other People's Smoke (Secondhand Smoke) Harm My Health And My Child's Health?

Breathing other people's smoke make children and adults who do not smoke sick. There is no safe level of breathing others people's smoke.

- Pregnant women who breathe other people's cigarette smoke are more likely to have a baby who weighs less.

- Babies who breathe in other people's cigarette smoke are more likely to have ear infections and more frequent asthma attacks.

- Babies who breathe in other people's cigarette smoke are more likely to die from SIDS. SIDS is an infant death for which a cause of the death cannot be found.

In the United States, 58 million children and adults who do not smoke are exposed to other people's smoke. Almost 25 million children and adolescents aged 3–19 years, or about 4 out of 10 children in this age group, are exposed to other people's cigarette smoke. Home and vehicles are the places where children are most exposed to cigarette smoke, and a major location of smoke exposure for adults too. Also, people can be exposed to cigarette smoke in public places, restaurants, and at work.

What Can You Do To Avoid Other People's Smoke?

There is no safe level of exposure to cigarette smoke. Breathing even a little smoke can be harmful. The only way to fully protect yourself and your loved ones from the dangers of other people's smoke is through 100 percent smoke-free environments.

You can protect yourself and your family by

- Making your home and car smoke-free.

- Asking people not to smoke around you and your children.

- Making sure that your children's daycare center or school is smoke-free.

- Choosing restaurants and other businesses that are smoke-free. Thanking businesses for being smoke-free.

- Teaching children to stay away from other people's smoke.

- Avoiding all smoke. If you or your children have respiratory conditions, if you have heart disease, or if you are pregnant, the dangers are greater for you.

- Learn as much as you can by talking to your doctor, nurse, or healthcare provider about the dangers of other people's smoke.

Chapter 28
Caffeine Use During Pregnancy

Pregnancy often means changes in diet, as well as other routines and habits, in order to ensure your own health and that of your baby. And one piece of diet advice that comes up frequently is to limit or eliminate the use of caffeine while you're pregnant. But after many decades of scientific study and observation, there's still no definitive answer about exactly how much caffeine—if any—is really safe for pregnant women.

> According to the U.S. Department of Health and Human Services (HHS), in addition to limiting caffeine intake during pregnancy, breastfeeding mothers should also reduce the amount they consume: "Drinking a moderate amount (up to 1 to 2 cups a day) of coffee or other caffeinated beverages does not cause a problem for most breastfeeding babies. But too much caffeine can cause a baby to be fussy or not sleep well."
>
> *(Source: "Breastfeeding And Everyday Life," U.S. Department of Health and Human Services (HHS).)*

What Is Caffeine And What Does It Do?

Caffeine is a naturally occurring substance found in the seeds and leaves of more than 60 plants. It's typically consumed in products like coffee, tea, colas and other soft drinks, chocolate, energy drinks, pain relievers, and other over-the-counter medications. It's a stimulant, so many people use it to wake up, stay awake, or feel more alert. According to the U.S. Food and Drug Administration (FDA), 80 percent of U.S. adults consume caffeine every day, with an average intake of 200mg, about the amount in an eight-ounce cup of coffee or four colas. It's

"Caffeine Use During Pregnancy," © 2017 Omnigraphics. Reviewed March 2017.

classified as a drug because of its effects on the brain and central nervous system. For example, the FDA says it can:

- make you jittery and shaky

- make it hard to fall asleep and stay asleep

- make your heart beat faster

- cause an uneven heart rhythm

- raise your blood pressure

- cause headaches, nervousness, and/or dizziness

- make you dehydrated

- make you dependent on it so you need more to get the same effect

> In addition to caffeine, coffee and tea also contain compounds that make it more difficult for the body to absorb iron. And since pregnant women already tend to have trouble getting enough iron, that's one more reason to reduce the consumption of these drinks during pregnancy.

What Are The Effects Of Caffeine During Pregnancy?

The first thing to understand is that when you ingest caffeine during pregnancy, you're passing the substance along to your fetus. Caffeine has the ability to cross the placenta easily, and the speed at which it metabolizes slows down during pregnancy, which means it stays in your system longer. In addition, fetuses tend to eliminate caffeine even more slowly, meaning their levels could remain even higher than the mother's.

The effects of caffeine on humans during pregnancy are not well known, despite a multitude of studies. Many have turned out inconclusive, and some have contradicted others. But many medical experts are concerned about animal studies that have shown that caffeine can cause:

- reduced fertility

- birth defects

- premature labor

- preterm delivery

- increased risk of low-birth weight offspring

It is worth noting, however, that in many of these tests, the pregnant animals were given much higher doses of caffeine, by body weight, than most people would ever ingest.

One of the biggest concerns about caffeine for pregnant women is that it might increase the risk of miscarriage. But this is still under investigation and being debated after a number of studies resulted in conflicting results. For example, one study found that women who consume 200mg or more of caffeine daily are twice as likely to have a miscarriage as those who don't consume any caffeine, while another study in the same year showed no increased risk of miscarriage among women who drank 220 to 350mg per day. One of the most extensive recent studies on the subject, published in the journal *Human Reproduction*, determined that caffeine consumption "during early pregnancy was associated with a small increased risk" of miscarriage, but the researchers could not establish a "dose-response relation" between caffeine and a higher risk of miscarriage. So the debate continues.

What To Do?

In spite of the conflicting evidence, one thing is certain: most experts recommend at least reducing your caffeine intake during pregnancy and some recommend eliminating it entirely. The March of Dimes, the American College of Obstetricians and Gynecologists (ACOG), and the Mayo Clinic all suggest limiting your caffeine intake to 200mg per day or less—at least until more conclusive studies are done. Below are some examples of the amount of caffeine in various common products:

- Brewed coffee (8oz.): 95–200mg

- Brewed decaffeinated coffee (8oz.): 2–12mg

- Instant coffee (8oz.): 27–173mg

- Espresso (1oz.): 47–75mg

- Latte or mocha (8oz.): 63–175mg

- Black tea (8oz.): 14–70mg

- Black decaffeinated tea (8oz.): 0–12mg

- Green tea (8oz.): 24–45mg

- Instant iced tea (8oz.): 11–47mg

- Bottled iced tea (8oz.): 5–40mg

- Cola (12oz.): 35–40mg

- Energy drinks (8oz.): 45–100mg

- Hot chocolate (8oz.): 3–15mg

- Milk chocolate (1.5oz. bar): 11mg

- Dark chocolate (1.5oz. bar): 31mg

- Chocolate pudding (5oz.): 9mg

- Chocolate cake (3oz.): 36mg

- Coffee ice cream or frozen yogurt (8oz.): 50–60mg

- Vitamin energy water (20oz.): 45–150mg

- Over-the-counter pain relievers (1 tablet): 30–200mg

> Various herbal products can also contain caffeine. Some of these include guarana, yerba mate, kola nut and green tea extract. Unlike other medications, the FDA does not require manufacturers to specify caffeine content on their labels, so most medical professionals recommend avoiding these products during pregnancy.

Note that caffeine amounts vary considerably depending on type and brand of the product, so read labels carefully or find a website that will give you more specific information. But this should give you an idea of what to expect as you work on restricting your caffeine intake.

References

1. "Caffeine During Pregnancy," Babycenter.com, January 2016.

2. "Caffeine in Pregnancy," Marchofdimes.org, October 2015.

3. "Caffeine Intake During Pregnancy," Americanpregnancy.org, September 2, 2016.

4. Hahn, K.A., PhD, MPH, et.al. "Caffeine and Caffeinated Beverage Consumption and Risk of Spontaneous Abortion," *Human Reproduction*, May 2015.

5. Hey, Edmund. "Coffee and Pregnancy," NIH.gov, February 24, 2007.

6. "Medicines in My Home: Caffeine and Your Body," U.S. Food and Drug Administration, 2007.

Chapter 29
Illicit Drug Use During Pregnancy

When you are pregnant, it is important that you watch what you put into your body. Consumption of illegal drugs is not safe for the unborn baby or for the mother.

Studies have shown that consumption of illegal drugs during pregnancy can result in miscarriage, low birth weight, premature labor, placental abruption, fetal death, and even maternal death.

Marijuana

Common Slang Names

Pot, weed, grass and reefer

What Happens When A Pregnant Woman Smokes Marijuana?

Marijuana crosses the placenta to your baby. Marijuana, like cigarette smoke, contains toxins that keep your baby from getting the proper supply of oxygen that he or she needs to grow.

How Can Marijuana Affect The Baby?

Studies of marijuana in pregnancy are inconclusive, because many women who smoke marijuana also use tobacco and alcohol. Smoking marijuana increases the levels of carbon monoxide and carbon dioxide in the blood, which reduces the oxygen supply to the baby. Smoking marijuana during pregnancy can increase the chance of miscarriage, low birth weight, premature births, developmental delays, and behavioral and learning problems.

About This Chapter: Text in this chapter is excerpted from "Using Illegal Drugs During Pregnancy," © 2017 American Pregnancy Association. Reprinted with permission.

What If I Smoked Marijuana Before I Knew I Was Pregnant?

According to Dr. Richard S. Abram, author of Will it Hurt the Baby, "occasional use of marijuana during the first trimester is unlikely to cause birth defects." Once you are aware you are pregnant, you should stop smoking. Doing this will decrease the chance of harming your baby.

Cocaine

Common Slang Names

Bump, toot, C, coke, crack, flake, snow, and candy

What Happens When A Pregnant Woman Consumes Cocaine?

Cocaine crosses the placenta and enters your baby's circulation. The elimination of cocaine is slower in a fetus than in an adult. This means that cocaine remains in the baby's body much longer than it does in your body.

How Can Cocaine Affect My Baby?

According to the Organization of Teratology Information Services (OTIS), during the early months of pregnancy cocaine exposure may increase the risk of miscarriage. Later in pregnancy, cocaine use can cause placental abruption, which can lead to severe bleeding, pre-term birth, and fetal death. OTIS also states that the risk of birth defects appears to be greater when the mother has used cocaine frequently during pregnancy.

According to the American Congress of Obstetricians and Gynecology (ACOG), women who use cocaine during their pregnancy have a 25 percent increased chance of premature labor. Babies born to mothers who use cocaine throughout their pregnancy may also have a smaller head and be growth restricted.

Babies who are exposed to cocaine later in pregnancy may be born dependent and suffer from withdrawal symptoms such as tremors, sleeplessness, muscle spasms, and feeding difficulties. Some experts believe that learning difficulties may result as the child gets older. Defects of the genitals, kidneys, and brain are also possible.

What If I Consumed Cocaine Before I Knew I Was Pregnant?

There have not been any conclusive studies done on single doses of cocaine during pregnancy. Birth defects and other side effects are usually a result of prolonged use, but because studies are inconclusive, it is best to avoid cocaine altogether. Cocaine is a very addictive drug and experimentation often leads to abuse of the drug.

Heroin

Common Slang Names

Horse, smack, junk, and H-stuff

What Happens When A Pregnant Woman Uses Heroin?

Heroin is a very addictive drug that crosses the placenta to the baby. Because this drug is so addictive, the unborn baby can become dependent on the drug.

How Can Heroin Affect My Baby?

Using heroin during pregnancy increases the chance of premature birth, low birth weight, breathing difficulties, low blood sugar (hypoglycemia), bleeding within the brain (intracranial hemorrhage), and infant death. Babies can also be born addicted to heroin and can suffer from withdrawal symptoms. Withdrawal symptoms include irritability, convulsions, diarrhea, fever, sleep abnormalities, and joint stiffness. Mothers who inject narcotics are more susceptible to HIV, which can be passed to their unborn children.

What If I Am Addicted To Heroin And I Am Pregnant?

Treating an addiction to heroin can be complicated, especially when you are pregnant. Your healthcare provider may prescribe methadone as a form of treatment. It is best that you communicate with your healthcare provider, so he or she can provide the best treatment for you and your baby.

PCP And LSD

What Happens When A Pregnant Woman Takes PCP And LSD?

Phencyclidine (PCP) and Lysergic acid diethylamide (LSD) are hallucinogens. Both PCP and LSD users can behave violently, which may harm the baby if the mother hurts herself.

How Can PCP And LSD Affect My Baby?

PCP use during pregnancy can lead to low birth weight, poor muscle control, brain damage, and withdrawal syndrome if used frequently. Withdrawal symptoms include lethargy, alternating with tremors. LSD can lead to birth defects if used frequently.

What If I Experimented With LSD Or PCP Before I Knew I Was Pregnant?

No conclusive studies have been done on one time use effects of these drugs on the fetus. It is best not to experiment if you are trying to get pregnant or think you might be pregnant.

Methamphetamine

Common Slang Names

Meth, speed, crystal, glass, and crank

What Happens When A Pregnant Woman Takes Methamphetamine?

Methamphetamine is chemically related to amphetamine, which causes the heart rate of the mother and baby to increase.

How Can Methamphetamine Affect My Baby?

Taking methamphetamine during pregnancy can result in problems similar to those seen with the use of cocaine in pregnancy. The use of speed can cause the baby to get less oxygen, which can lead to low birth weight. Methamphetamine can also increase the likelihood of premature labor, miscarriage, and placental abruption. Babies can be born addicted to methamphetamine and suffer withdrawal symptoms that include tremors, sleeplessness, muscle spasms, and feeding difficulties. Some experts believe that learning difficulties may result as the child gets older.

What If I Experimented With Methamphetamine Before I Knew I Was Pregnant?

There have not been any significant studies done on the effect of one time use of methamphetamine during pregnancy. It is best not to experiment if you are trying to get pregnant or think you might be pregnant.

Chapter 30

Environmental Risks And Pregnancy

Climate change threatens human health, including mental health, and access to clean air, safe drinking water, nutritious food, and shelter. Everyone is affected by climate change at some point in their lives. Some people are more affected by climate change than others because of factors like where they live; their age, health, income, and occupation; and how they go about their day-to-day life.

Most women have healthy pregnancies and healthy babies. However, climate change can worsen environmental hazards that threaten the health of pregnant women and increase health risks for the baby, such as:

- **Low weight of the baby at birth.** If a baby weighs less than 5.5 pounds at birth, there may be lasting effects on health.

- **Preterm birth.** Labor that starts before 37 weeks of pregnancy is considered preterm, and may lead to health problems.

Air pollutants can cause respiratory illness in pregnant women and also lead to low birth weight or preterm birth. Climate change worsens air quality because warming temperatures make it easier for ground-level ozone to form. Changing weather patterns and more intense and frequent wildfires also raise the amount of pollution, dust, and smoke in the air.

About This Chapter: Text in this chapter begins with excerpts from "Climate Change And The Health Of Pregnant Women," U.S. Environmental Protection Agency (EPA), May 2016; Text beginning with the heading "Mercury And The Body" is excerpted from "Mercury," Centers for Disease Control and Prevention (CDC), October 14, 2015; Text under the heading "Are You Pregnant?" is excerpted from "Pregnant Women," Centers for Disease Control and Prevention (CDC), June 15, 2013. Reviewed March 2017.

Climate change will also cause extreme heat events to become more frequent and to become more frequent and to become more frequent and in pregnant women. Dehydration early in pregnancy can affect the baby's growth and later in pregnancy can cause preterm birth.

Under a changing climate, hurricane intensity and rainfall are expected to increase and floods may occur more often or be more severe. These types of extreme weather events increase health risks to pregnant women. Poor nutrition and diarrhea from contaminated water or food have been linked to negative birth outcomes such as low birth weight. Floods can lead to an increase in exposure to toxins and mold. Severe weather events may damage homes, other buildings, and roads or require evacuations, which can make it more difficult for pregnant women to get the specialized healthcare they need.

Physical outcomes related to environmental hazards are not the only concern for pregnant women. Pregnant women and women who have recently given birth (postpartum) are at an increased risk for severe stress and other negative mental health outcomes due to weather-related disasters associated with climate change. Severe maternal stress can increase risk of negative outcomes such as preterm birth.

Mercury And The Body

> Exposure to some toxic substances—including lead, mercury, arsenic, cadmium, pesticides, solvents, and household chemicals—can increase the risk of miscarriage, preterm birth, and other pregnancy complications. These and other environmental toxins can also harm the developing bodies of fetuses and infants. Women who are pregnant or nursing or who plan to become pregnant should take special care to avoid exposure to certain chemicals.
>
> (Source: "The Environment And Women's Health Fact Sheet," Office on Women's Health (OWH), U.S. Department of Health and Human Services (HHS).)

Oral exposure to mercury results in very small amounts getting into your body.

When you swallow small amounts of metallic mercury, for example, from a broken oral thermometer, virtually none (less than 0.01%) of the mercury will enter your body through the stomach or intestines, unless they are diseased. Even when a larger amount of metal mercury (a half of a tablespoon, about 204 grams) was swallowed by one person, very little entered the body. When you breathe in mercury vapors, however, most (about 80%) of the mercury enters your bloodstream directly from your lungs, and then rapidly goes to other parts of your body, including the brain and kidneys. Once in your body, metallic mercury can stay for weeks or months. When metallic mercury enters the brain, it is readily converted to an inorganic form and is "trapped" in the brain for a long time. Metallic mercury in the blood of a pregnant woman can enter her developing child. Most of the metallic mercury will accumulate in your kidneys, but some metallic mercury can also accumulate in the brain. Most of the metallic mercury absorbed into the body eventually leaves in the urine and feces, while smaller amounts leave the body in the exhaled breath.

Inorganic mercury compounds like mercurous chloride and mercuric chloride are white powders and do not generally vaporize at room temperatures like elemental mercury will. If they are inhaled, they are not expected to enter your body as easily as inhaled metallic mercury vapor. When inorganic mercury compounds are swallowed, generally less than 10 percent is absorbed through the intestinal tract; however, up to 40 percent may enter the body through the stomach and intestines in some instances. Some inorganic mercury can enter your body through the skin, but only a small amount will pass through your skin compared to the amount that gets into your body from swallowing inorganic mercury. Once inorganic mercury enters the body and gets into the bloodstream, it moves to many different tissues. Inorganic mercury leaves your body in the urine or feces over a period of several weeks or months. A small amount of the inorganic mercury can be changed in your body to metallic mercury and leave in the breath as a mercury vapor. Inorganic mercury accumulates mostly in the kidneys and does not enter the brain as easily as metallic mercury. Inorganic mercury compounds also do not move as easily from the blood of a pregnant woman to her developing child. In a nursing woman, some of the inorganic mercury in her body will pass into her breast milk.

Methylmercury is the form of mercury most easily absorbed through the gastrointestinal tract (about 95 percent absorbed). After you eat fish or other foods that are contaminated with methylmercury, the methylmercury enters your bloodstream easily and goes rapidly to other parts of your body. Only small amounts of methylmercury enter the bloodstream directly through the skin, but other forms of organic mercury (in particular dimethylmercury) can rapidly enter the body through the skin. Organic mercury compounds may evaporate slowly at room temperature and may enter your body easily if you breathe in the vapors. Once organic mercury is in the bloodstream, it moves easily to most tissues and readily enters the brain. Methylmercury that is in the blood of a pregnant woman will easily move into the blood of the developing child and then into the child's brain and other tissues. Like metallic mercury, methylmercury can be changed by your body to inorganic mercury. When this happens in the brain, the mercury can remain there for a long time. When methylmercury does leave your body after you have been exposed, it leaves slowly over a period of several months, mostly as inorganic mercury in the feces. As with inorganic mercury, some of the methylmercury in a nursing woman's body will pass into her breast milk.

Mercury And Pregnant Women

Children are at risk of being exposed to mercury in a number of ways.

Some of these routes may include exposure to metallic mercury that is not safely contained, to mercury that may be brought home on work clothes or tools, or to methylmercury-contaminated foods. Methylmercury eaten or swallowed by a pregnant woman or metallic mercury that enters her body from breathing contaminated air can also pass into the developing child. Inorganic mercury and methylmercury can also pass from a mother's body into breast milk and into a nursing infant. The amount of mercury in the milk will vary, depending on the degree of exposure and the amount of mercury that enter the nursing woman's body. There are significant benefits to breastfeeding, so any concern that a nursing woman may have about mercury levels in her breast milk should be discussed with her doctor. Methylmercury can also accumulate in an unborn baby's blood to a concentration higher than the concentration in the mother.

In critical periods of development before they are born, and in the early months after birth, children and fetuses are particularly sensitive to the harmful effects of metallic mercury and methylmercury on the nervous system. Harmful developmental effects may occur when a pregnant woman is exposed to metallic mercury and some of the mercury is transferred into her developing child. Thus, women who are normally exposed to mercury vapors in the workplace (such as those working in thermometer/barometer or fluorescent light manufacturing or the chloralkali industry) should take measures to avoid mercury vapor exposures during pregnancy. Exposures to mercury vapors are relatively rare outside of the workplace, unless metallic mercury is present in the home.

Methylmercury is the form of mercury most commonly associated with a risk for developmental effects. Exposure can come from foods contaminated with mercury on the surface (for example, from seed grain treated with methylmercury to kill fungus) or from foods that contain toxic levels of methylmercury (as in some fish, wild game, and marine mammals). Mothers who are exposed to methylmercury and breast-feed their infant may also expose the child through the milk. The effects on the infant may be subtle or more pronounced, depending on the amount to which the fetus or young child was exposed. In cases in which the exposure was very small, some effects might not be apparent, such as small decreases in IQ or effects on the brain that may only be determined by the use of very sensitive neuropsychological testing. In instances in which the exposure is great, the effects may be more serious. In some such cases of mercury exposure involving serious exposure to the developing fetus, the effects are delayed. In such cases, the infant may be born apparently normal, but later show effects that may range from the infant being slower to reach developmental milestones, such as the age of first walking and talking, to more severe effects including brain damage with mental retardation, incoordination, and inability to move.

Other severe effects observed in children whose mothers were exposed to very toxic levels of mercury during pregnancy include eventual blindness, involuntary muscle contractions and seizures, muscle weakness, and inability to speak. It is important to remember, however, that the severity of these effects depends upon the level of mercury exposure and the time of exposure. The very severe effects just mentioned were reported in large-scale poisoning instances in which pregnant and nursing women were exposed to extremely high levels of methylmercury in contaminated grain used to make bread (in Iraq) or seafood (in Japan) sold to the general population.

Researchers are studying the potential for less serious developmental effects, including effects on a child's behavior and ability to learn, think, and solve problems that may result from eating lower levels of methylmercury in foods. A main source of exposure to methylmercury for the pregnant woman and the young child is from eating fish. Most fish purchased in the market in the United States do not have mercury levels that pose a risk to anyone, including pregnant women. Since mercury accumulates in the muscles of fish, larger fish that feed on smaller fish and live for long periods usually have larger concentrations of methylmercury than fish that feed on plants. For example, shark and swordfish normally contain the highest levels of mercury out of all ocean fish. Scientists have an ongoing debate about the value of fish in the diet versus any risk from increased exposure of pregnant women to methylmercury that may be in the fish. The safety of most fish sold commercially in the United States is regulated by the U.S. Food and Drug Administration (FDA). These fish pose no health risk to those who purchase and eat them. Only fish or wildlife containing relatively high levels of methylmercury are of concern.

Are You Pregnant?

Prevent Lead Poisoning. Start Now.

Lead poisoning is caused by breathing or swallowing lead. Lead can pass from a mother to her unborn baby.

Too much lead in your body can

- Put you at risk for miscarriage.

- Cause your baby to be born too early or too small.

- Hurt your baby's brain, kidneys, and nervous system.

- Cause your child to have learning or behavior problems.

Lead can be found in

- Paint and dust in older homes, especially dust from renovation or repairs.

- Candy, make up, glazed pots, and folk medicine made in other countries.

- Work like auto refinishing, construction, and plumbing.

- Soil and tap water.

Now Is The Time To Keep Your Baby Safe From Lead Poisoning. Here's What You Can Do:

1. **Watch out for lead in your home.**

   Most lead comes from paint in older homes. When old paint cracks and peels, it makes dangerous dust. The dust is so small you cannot see it. You can breathe in lead dust and not even know it.

   Home repairs like sanding or scraping paint can make dangerous lead dust. You should not be in the house while someone is cleaning up after renovations, painting, or remodeling a room with lead paint.

2. **Talk to your doctor.**

   Talk to your doctor about any medicines or vitamins you are taking. Some home remedies and dietary supplements may have lead in them. It is also important to tell your doctor about any cravings you have such as eating dirt or clay, because they may have lead in them.

3. **Avoid certain jobs or hobbies.**

   Some jobs or hobbies involve lead exposure. Such work includes construction or home renovation/repair in older homes, and battery manufacturing or recycling. Also, avoid take-home lead dust if a household member works with lead. It is a good idea to have the household member change into clean clothing before coming home. Keep work shoes outside and wash all work clothes separately from the rest of the family.

4. **Eat foods with calcium, iron, and vitamin C.**

   These foods may help protect you and your unborn baby.

   - Calcium is in milk, yogurt, cheese, and green leafy vegetables like spinach.

- Iron is in lean red meat, beans, cereals, and spinach.

- Vitamin C is in oranges, green and red peppers, broccoli, tomatoes, and juices.

Use caution when eating candies, spices, and other foods that have been brought into the country by travelers, especially if they appear to be noncommercial products.

5. **Store food properly.**

Some dishes may contain lead. It is important to store and serve your food properly.

- Avoid using imported lead-glazed ceramic pottery produced in cottage industries.

- Avoid using pewter or brass containers or utensils to cook, serve, or store food.

- Avoid using leaded crystal to serve or store beverages.

- Do not use dishes that are chipped or cracked.

Chapter 31
Zika And Pregnancy

What Is Zika?

Zika virus disease is caused by the Zika virus, which is spread to people primarily through the bite of an infected mosquito (*Aedes aegypti* and *Aedes albopictus*). The illness is usually mild with symptoms lasting up to a week, and many people do not have symptoms or will have only mild symptoms. However, Zika virus infection during pregnancy can cause a serious birth defect called microcephaly and other severe brain defects.

How Do People Get Infected With Zika?

Zika is spread to people primarily through the bite of an infected *Aedes* species mosquito (*Aedes aegypti* and *Aedes albopictus*). A pregnant woman can pass Zika to her fetus during pregnancy or around the time of birth. Also, a person with Zika can pass it to his or her sex partners. CDC encourages people who have traveled to or live in places with Zika to protect themselves by preventing mosquito bites and sexual transmission of Zika.

Should Pregnant Women Travel To Areas Where Zika Has Been Confirmed?

No. Pregnant women should not travel to any area with Zika. Travelers who go to places with outbreaks of Zika can be infected with Zika, and Zika infection during pregnancy can cause microcephaly and other severe fetal brain defects.

About This Chapter: This chapter includes text excerpted from "Questions About Zika," Centers for Disease Control and Prevention (CDC), October 17, 2016.

What Can People Do To Prevent Zika?

The best way to prevent Zika is to protect yourself and your family from mosquito bites:

- Use Environmental Protection Agency (EPA)-registered insect repellents

- Wear long-sleeved shirts and long pants

- Sleep under a mosquito bed net if air conditioned or screened rooms are not available or if sleeping outdoors.

Zika can be spread by a person infected with Zika to his or her sex partners. Condoms can reduce the chance of getting Zika from sex. Condoms include male and female condoms. To be effective, condoms should be used from start to finish, every time during vaginal, anal, and oral sex and the sharing of sex toys. Not having sex eliminates the risk of getting Zika from sex. Pregnant couples with a partner who traveled to or lives in an area with Zika should use condoms every time they have sex or not have sex during the pregnancy.

What Are The Symptoms Of Zika Virus Disease?

The most common symptoms of Zika virus disease are fever, rash, joint pain, and red eyes. Other symptoms include muscle pain and headache. Many people infected with Zika won't have symptoms or will have mild symptoms, which can last for several days to a week.

How Is Zika Diagnosed?

To diagnose Zika, your doctor will ask you about recent travel and symptoms you may have, and collect blood or urine to test for Zika or similar viruses.

Can Someone Who Returned From An Area With Zika Get Tested For The Virus?

Zika virus testing is performed at Centers for Disease Control and Prevention (CDC) and some state and territorial health departments. See your doctor if you have Zika symptoms and have recently been in an area with Zika. Your doctor may order tests to look for Zika or similar viruses like dengue and chikungunya.

What Should Pregnant Women Who Have Recently Traveled To An Area With Zika Do?

Pregnant women who have recently traveled to an area with Zika should talk to their doctor about their travel, even if they don't feel sick. Pregnant women should see a doctor if they have any Zika symptoms during their trip or within 2 weeks after traveling. All pregnant women can protect themselves by avoiding travel to an area with Zika, preventing mosquito bites, and following recommended precautions against getting Zika through sex.

I Am Not Pregnant, But Will My Future Pregnancies Be At Risk If I Am Infected With Zika Virus?

Currently, there is no evidence that a woman who has recovered from Zika virus infection (the virus has cleared her body) will have Zika-related pregnancy complications in the future. Based on information about similar infections, once a person has been infected with Zika virus and has cleared the virus, he or she is likely to be protected from future Zika infections.

If you're thinking about having a baby in the near future and you or your partner live in or traveled to an area with Zika, talk with your doctor or other healthcare provider. Men who have traveled to an areas with Zika or who have had Zika infection should wait at least 6 months after travel (or 6 months after symptoms started if they get sick) before trying to conceive with their partner. Women should wait at least 8 weeks after travel (or 8 weeks after symptoms started if they get sick) before trying to get pregnant.

I Was In A Place With Zika Recently. How Long Do I Need To Wait After Returning To Get Pregnant?

Men who have traveled to a place with Zika should wait at least 6 months after travel (or 6 months after symptoms started if they get sick) before trying to conceive with their partner. Women should wait at least 8 weeks after travel (or 8 weeks after symptoms started if they get sick) before trying to get pregnant. The waiting period is longer for men because Zika stays in semen longer than in other body fluids.

Part Four
High-Risk Pregnancies And Pregnancy Complications

Chapter 32

High-Risk Pregnancy

A high-risk pregnancy refers to anything that puts the mother or fetus at increased risk for poor health during pregnancy or childbirth. A pregnancy is considered high risk if the mother has chronic health conditions such as high blood pressure or diabetes, or if she weighs too much or too little. Any pregnancy where complications are more likely than normal is considered a high-risk pregnancy.

What Are The Factors That Put A Pregnancy At Risk?

The factors that place a pregnancy at risk can be divided into four categories:

1. Existing Health Conditions

2. Age

3. Lifestyle Factors

4. Conditions of Pregnancy

Existing Health Conditions

- **High blood pressure.** Even though high blood pressure can be risky for mother and fetus, many women with high blood pressure have healthy pregnancies and healthy children. Uncontrolled high blood pressure, however, can lead to damage to the mother's kidneys and increases the risk for low birth weight or preeclampsia.

About This Chapter: This chapter includes text excerpted from "High-Risk Pregnancy: Condition Information," *Eunice Kennedy Shriver* National Institute of Child Health and Human Development (NICHD), July 17, 2012. Reviewed March 2017.

- **Polycystic ovary syndrome.** Polycystic ovary syndrome (PCOS) is a disorder that can interfere with a woman's ability to get and stay pregnant. PCOS may result in higher rates of miscarriage (the spontaneous loss of the fetus before 20 weeks of pregnancy), gestational diabetes, preeclampsia, and premature delivery.

- **Diabetes.** It is important for women with diabetes to manage their blood sugar levels before getting pregnant. High blood sugar levels can cause birth defects during the first few weeks of pregnancy, often before women even know they are pregnant. Controlling blood sugar levels and taking a multivitamin with 40 micrograms of folic acid every day can help reduce this risk.

- **Kidney disease.** Women with kidney disease often have difficulty getting pregnant, and any pregnancy is at significant risk for miscarriage. Pregnant women with kidney disease require additional treatments, changes in diet and medication, and frequent visits to their healthcare provider.

- **Autoimmune disease.** Autoimmune diseases include conditions such as lupus and multiple sclerosis. Some autoimmune diseases can increase women's risk for problems during pregnancy. For example, lupus can increase the risk for preterm birth and stillbirth. Some women may find that their symptoms improve during pregnancy, while others experience flare ups and other challenges. Certain medications to treat autoimmune diseases may be harmful to the fetus as well.

- **Thyroid disease.** Uncontrolled thyroid disease, such as an overactive or underactive thyroid (small gland in the neck that makes hormones that regulate the heart rate and blood pressure) can cause problems for the fetus, such as heart failure, poor weight gain, and birth defects.

- **Infertility.** Several studies have found that women who take drugs that increase the chances of pregnancy are significantly more likely to have pregnancy complications than those who get pregnant without assistance. These complications often involve the placenta (the organ linking the fetus and the mother) and vaginal bleeding.

- **Obesity.** Obesity can make a pregnancy more difficult, increasing a woman's chance of developing diabetes during pregnancy, which can contribute to difficult births. On the other hand, some women weigh too little for their own health and the health of their growing fetus.

- **HIV/AIDS.** HIV damages cells of the immune system, making it difficult to fight infections and certain cancers. Women can pass the virus to their fetus during pregnancy;

transmission also can occur during labor and giving birth or through breastfeeding. Fortunately, effective treatments exist to reduce the spread of HIV from the mother to her fetus, newborn, or infant. Women with very low viral loads may be able to have a vaginal delivery with a low risk of transmission. An option for pregnant women with higher viral loads (measurement of the amount of active HIV in the blood) is a Cesarean delivery, which reduces the risk of passing HIV to the infant during labor and delivery. Early and regular prenatal care is important. Women who take medication to treat their HIV and have a Cesarean delivery can reduce the risk of transmission to 2 percent.

Age

- **Teen pregnancy.** Pregnant teens are more likely to develop high blood pressure and anemia (lack of healthy red blood cells), and go into labor earlier than women who are older. Teens also may be exposed to a sexually transmitted disease or infection that could affect their pregnancy. Teens may be less likely to get prenatal care or to make ongoing appointments with healthcare providers during the pregnancy to evaluate risks, ensure they are staying healthy, and understand what medications and drugs they can use.

Lifestyle Factors

- **Alcohol use.** Alcohol consumed during pregnancy passes directly to the fetus through the umbilical cord. The Centers for Disease Control and Prevention recommend that women avoid alcoholic beverages during pregnancy or when they are trying to get pregnant. During pregnancy, women who drink are more likely to have a miscarriage or stillbirth. Other risks to the fetus include a higher chance of having birth defects and fetal alcohol spectrum disorder (FASD). FASD is the technical name for the group of fetal disorders that have been associated with drinking alcohol during pregnancy. It causes abnormal facial features, short stature and low body weight, hyperactivity disorder, intellectual disabilities, and vision or hearing problems.

- **Cigarette smoking.** Smoking during pregnancy puts the fetus at risk for preterm birth, certain birth defects, and sudden infant death syndrome (SIDS). Secondhand smoke also puts a woman and her developing fetus at increased risk for health problems.

Conditions Of Pregnancy

- **Multiple gestation.** Pregnancy with twins, triplets, or more, referred to as a multiple gestation, increases the risk of infants being born prematurely (before 37 weeks of pregnancy). Having infants after age 30 and taking fertility drugs both have been associated with multiple births. Having three or more infants increases the chance that a woman will need to have the infants delivered by Cesarean section. Twins and triplets are more likely to be smaller for their size than infants of singleton births. If infants of multiple gestation are born prematurely, they are more likely to have difficulty breathing.

- **Gestational diabetes.** Gestational diabetes, also known as gestational diabetes mellitus, GDM, or diabetes during pregnancy, is diabetes that first develops when a woman is pregnant. Many women can have healthy pregnancies if they manage their diabetes, following a diet and treatment plan from their healthcare provider. Uncontrolled gestational diabetes increases the risk for preterm labor and delivery, preeclampsia, and high blood pressure.

- **Preeclampsia and eclampsia.** Preeclampsia is a syndrome marked by a sudden increase in the blood pressure of a pregnant woman after the 20th week of pregnancy. It can affect the mother's kidneys, liver, and brain. When left untreated, the condition can be fatal for the mother and/or the fetus and result in long-term health problems. Eclampsia is a more severe form of preeclampsia, marked by seizures and coma in the mother.

How Many People Are At Risk Of Having A High-Risk Pregnancy?

The more risk factors a woman has, the more likely she and her fetus will be at risk during pregnancy and birth. Statistics are available for some risk factors:

- **High blood pressure.** According to statistics collected by the National Heart, Lung, and Blood Institute (NHLBI), about 6 to 8 percent of pregnant women in the United States have high blood pressure. About 70 percent of them are women who are pregnant for the first time.

- **Preeclampsia.** Preeclampsia affects an estimated 3 to 5 percent of pregnancies in the United States, and 5 to 10 percent of all pregnancies globally. The majority occur at term.

- **Gestational diabetes.** According to the Centers for Disease Control and Prevention (CDC), gestational diabetes affects 2 to 10 percent of pregnancies.

How Is High-Risk Pregnancy Diagnosed?

Good prenatal care will help to identify the potential for high-risk pregnancy. Healthcare providers will ask a woman about her medical history and will perform assessments to determine whether she is likely to experience a high-risk pregnancy based on her risk factors. Ongoing monitoring of physical health and personal habits will help a healthcare provider identify problems that develop during pregnancy.

A woman with a high-risk pregnancy will also likely receive care from a special team of healthcare providers throughout the pregnancy to ensure that she carries the fetus or fetuses to term.

Can A High-Risk Pregnancy Be Prevented?

Staying healthy is one of the best ways to lower the risk of having a difficult pregnancy. Many healthcare providers recommend that women who are thinking about becoming pregnant get evaluated to make sure they are in good preconception health. During pregnancy, there are also steps a woman can take to reduce the risk of certain problems:

- Take at least 400 micrograms of folic acid (a type of vitamin B) every day before and during pregnancy.
- Get proper immunizations.
- Maintain a healthy weight; eat a good diet; get regular physical exercise; and avoid smoking, alcohol, or drug use.
- Start prenatal care appointments early during pregnancy and visit a health provider for regularly scheduled appointments throughout the pregnancy.

What Are Common Treatments For High-Risk Pregnancy?

For women who are diagnosed with a high-risk pregnancy, treatment varies depending on the risk factors.

High Blood Pressure

Some changes to high blood pressure medication may be necessary during pregnancy. A healthcare provider can also offer advice about the best way to keep blood pressure under control. Suggestions may include recommendations to limit salt intake and get regular exercise.

Gestational Diabetes

Gestational diabetes, or developing diabetes during pregnancy, increases the risk of pregnancy complications. However, many women have healthy pregnancies and healthy infants because they follow a healthcare provider's recommended diet and treatment plan. A woman diagnosed with gestational diabetes should:

- **Know her blood sugar level and keep it under control.** A women diagnosed with gestational diabetes can track her own blood sugar levels by testing several times a day.

- **Eat a healthy diet.** A low carbohydrate diet with meals spread throughout the day helps to keep blood sugar under control. Healthcare providers will offer advice for developing a plan with the best diet for each individual.

- **Keep a healthy weight.** The amount of weight gain that is healthy for a woman will depend on how much she weighed before pregnancy. It is important to track both overall weight gain and the weekly rate of weight gain.

- **Keep daily records of diet, physical activity, and glucose level.** A woman with gestational diabetes should write down her blood sugar numbers, physical activity, and everything she eats and drinks in a daily record book.

Some women with gestational diabetes will also need to take medicine, such as an oral hypoglycemic tablet or insulin to help manage their diabetes.

HIV Treatment

HIV infection can be passed from a mother to her fetus as well as during childbirth and breastfeeding, but treatment can prevent transmission.

High-Risk Pregnancy: Other FAQs
How Do I Know If I Have Or Will Have A High-Risk Pregnancy?

If you are thinking about getting pregnant or are already pregnant, visit your healthcare provider. He or she will check your medical history and run tests to determine whether you are likely to have a high-risk pregnancy. Your healthcare provider will help you come up with a plan for reducing the risks while you are pregnant.

How Can I Best Take Care Of Myself And My Fetus During My Pregnancy?

You can take care of yourself and your fetus during pregnancy by eating healthy; avoiding drugs, smoking, and alcohol; exercising regularly; getting good prenatal care; and following your healthcare provider's recommendations.

If I Get Gestational Diabetes, Will I Still Have Diabetes After The Infant Is Born?

If you develop diabetes during pregnancy, typically, you do not continue to have diabetes after delivery. However, gestational diabetes can raise a woman's risk of developing diabetes later in life. A study led by *Eunice Kennedy Shriver* National Institute of Child Health and Human Development (NICHD) found that, among women who have had gestational diabetes, following a healthy diet after pregnancy may help prevent type 2 diabetes from developing.

Chapter 33
Genetic Testing

What Is Genetic Testing?

Genetic testing is a type of medical test that identifies changes in chromosomes, genes, or proteins. The results of a genetic test can confirm or rule out a suspected genetic condition or help determine a person's chance of developing or passing on a genetic disorder. More than 1,000 genetic tests are currently in use, and more are being developed.

Several methods can be used for genetic testing:

- Molecular genetic tests (or gene tests) study single genes or short lengths of deoxyribonucleic acid (DNA) to identify variations or mutations that lead to a genetic disorder.

- Chromosomal genetic tests analyze whole chromosomes or long lengths of DNA to see if there are large genetic changes, such as an extra copy of a chromosome, that cause a genetic condition.

- Biochemical genetic tests study the amount or activity level of proteins; abnormalities in either can indicate changes to the DNA that result in a genetic disorder.

Genetic testing is voluntary. Because testing has benefits as well as limitations and risks, the decision about whether to be tested is a personal and complex one. A geneticist or genetic counselor can help by providing information about the pros and cons of the test and discussing the social and emotional aspects of testing.

About This Chapter: This chapter includes text excerpted from "Genetic Testing," Genetics Home Reference (GHR), National Institutes of Health (NIH), February 7, 2017.

What Are The Types Of Genetic Tests?

Genetic testing can provide information about a person's genes and chromosomes. Available types of testing include:

- Carrier Testing
- Diagnostic Testing
- Forensic Testing
- Newborn Screening
- Predictive And Presymptomatic Testing
- Preimplantation Testing
- Prenatal Testing

How Is Genetic Testing Done?

Once a person decides to proceed with genetic testing, a medical geneticist, primary care doctor, specialist, or nurse practitioner can order the test. Genetic testing is often done as part of a genetic consultation.

Genetic tests are performed on a sample of blood, hair, skin, amniotic fluid (the fluid that surrounds a fetus during pregnancy), or other tissue. For example, a procedure called a buccal smear uses a small brush or cotton swab to collect a sample of cells from the inside surface of the cheek. The sample is sent to a laboratory where technicians look for specific changes in chromosomes, DNA, or proteins, depending on the suspected disorder. The laboratory reports the test results in writing to a person's doctor or genetic counselor, or directly to the patient if requested.

Newborn screening tests are done on a small blood sample, which is taken by pricking the baby's heel. Unlike other types of genetic testing, a parent will usually only receive the result if it is positive. If the test result is positive, additional testing is needed to determine whether the baby has a genetic disorder.

What Do The Results Of Genetic Tests Mean?

The results of genetic tests are not always straightforward, which often makes them challenging to interpret and explain. Therefore, it is important for patients and their families to ask questions about the potential meaning of genetic test results both before and after the test is performed. When interpreting test results, healthcare professionals consider a person's medical history, family history, and the type of genetic test that was done.

Table 33.1. Common Prenatal Tests

Test	What It Is	How It Is Done
Amniocentesis	This test can diagnosis certain birth defects, including: • Down syndrome • Cystic fibrosis • Spina bifida It is performed at 14 to 20 weeks. It may be suggested for couples at higher risk for genetic disorders. It also provides DNA for paternity testing.	A thin needle is used to draw out a small amount of amniotic fluid and cells from the sac surrounding the fetus. The sample is sent to a lab for testing.
Biophysical profile (BPP)	This test is used in the third trimester to monitor the overall health of the baby and to help decide if the baby should be delivered early.	BPP involves an ultrasound exam along with a nonstress test. The BPP looks at the baby's breathing, movement, muscle tone, heart rate, and the amount of amniotic fluid.
Chorionic villus sampling (CVS)	A test done at 10 to 13 weeks to diagnose certain birth defects, including: • Chromosomal disorders, including Down syndrome • Genetic disorders, such as cystic fibrosis CVS may be suggested for couples at higher risk for genetic disorders. It also provides DNA for paternity testing.	A needle removes a small sample of cells from the placenta to be tested.
First trimester screen	A screening test done at 11 to 14 weeks to detect higher risk of: • Chromosomal disorders, including Down syndrome and trisomy 18 • Other problems, such as heart defects It also can reveal multiple births. Based on test results, your doctor may suggest other tests to diagnose a disorder.	This test involves both a blood test and an ultrasound exam called nuchal translucency screening. The blood test measures the levels of certain substances in the mother's blood. The ultrasound exam measures the thickness at the back of the baby's neck. This information, combined with the mother's age, help doctors determine risk to the fetus.

Table 33.1. Continued

Test	What It Is	How It Is Done
Glucose challenge screening	A screening test done at 26 to 28 weeks to determine the mother's risk of gestational diabetes. Based on test results, your doctor may suggest a glucose tolerance test.	First, you consume a special sugary drink from your doctor. A blood sample is taken one hour later to look for high blood sugar levels.
Glucose tolerance test	This test is done at 26 to 28 weeks to diagnose gestational diabetes.	Your doctor will tell you what to eat a few days before the test. Then, you cannot eat or drink anything but sips of water for 14 hours before the test. Your blood is drawn to test your "fasting blood glucose level." Then, you will consume a sugary drink. Your blood will be tested every hour for three hours to see how well your body processes sugar.
Group B streptococcus infection	This test is done at 36 to 37 weeks to look for bacteria that can cause pneumonia or serious infection in newborn.	A swab is used to take cells from your vagina and rectum to be tested.
Maternal serum screen (also called quad screen, triple screen, triple test, triple screen, multiple marker screen, or AFP)	A screening test done at 15 to 20 weeks to detect higher risk of: • Chromosomal disorders, including Down syndrome and trisomy 18 • Neural tube defects, such as spina bifida Based on test results, your doctor may suggest other tests to diagnose a disorder.	Blood is drawn to measure the levels of certain substances in the mother's blood.
Nonstress test (NST)	This test is performed after 28 weeks to monitor your baby's health. It can show signs of fetal distress, such as your baby not getting enough oxygen.	A belt is placed around the mother's belly to measure the baby's heart rate in response to its own movements.

Table 33.1. Continued

Test	What It Is	How It Is Done
Ultrasound exam	An ultrasound exam can be performed at any point during the pregnancy. Ultrasound exams are not routine. But it is not uncommon for women to have a standard ultrasound exam between 18 and 20 weeks to look for signs of problems with the baby's organs and body systems and confirm the age of the fetus and proper growth. It also might be able to tell the sex of your baby. Ultrasound exam is also used as part of the first trimester screen and biophysical profile (BPP). Based on exam results, your doctor may suggest other tests or other types of ultrasound to help detect a problem.	Ultrasound uses sound waves to create a "picture" of your baby on a monitor. With a standard ultrasound, a gel is spread on your abdomen. A special tool is moved over your abdomen, which allows your doctor and you to view the baby on a monitor.
Urine test	A urine sample can look for signs of health problems, such as: • Urinary tract infection • Diabetes • Preeclampsia If your doctor suspects a problem, the sample might be sent to a lab for more in-depth testing.	You will collect a small sample of clean, midstream urine in a sterile plastic cup. Testing strips that look for certain substances in your urine are dipped in the sample. The sample also can be looked at under a microscope.

(Source: "Prenatal Care And Tests," Office on Women's Health (OWH), U.S. Department of Health and Human Services (HHS).)

A positive test result means that the laboratory found a change in a particular gene, chromosome, or protein of interest. Depending on the purpose of the test, this result may confirm a diagnosis, indicate that a person is a carrier of a particular genetic mutation, identify an increased risk of developing a disease (such as cancer) in the future, or suggest a need for further testing. Because family members have some genetic material in common, a positive test result may also have implications for certain blood relatives of the person undergoing testing. It is important to note that a positive result of a predictive or presymptomatic genetic test usually cannot establish the exact risk of developing a disorder. Also, health professionals typically cannot use a positive test result to predict the course or severity of a condition.

A negative test result means that the laboratory did not find a change in the gene, chromosome, or protein under consideration. This result can indicate that a person is not affected by a particular disorder, is not a carrier of a specific genetic mutation, or does not have an increased risk of developing a certain disease. It is possible, however, that the test missed a disease-causing genetic alteration because many tests cannot detect all genetic changes that can cause a particular disorder. Further testing may be required to confirm a negative result.

In some cases, a test result might not give any useful information. This type of result is called uninformative, indeterminate, inconclusive, or ambiguous. Uninformative test results sometimes occur because everyone has common, natural variations in their DNA, called polymorphisms, that do not affect health. If a genetic test finds a change in DNA that has not been associated with a disorder in other people, it can be difficult to tell whether it is a natural polymorphism or a disease-causing mutation. An uninformative result cannot confirm or rule out a specific diagnosis, and it cannot indicate whether a person has an increased risk of developing a disorder. In some cases, testing other affected and unaffected family members can help clarify this type of result.

What Are The Benefits Of Genetic Testing?

Genetic testing has potential benefits whether the results are positive or negative for a gene mutation. Test results can provide a sense of relief from uncertainty and help people make informed decisions about managing their healthcare. For example, a negative result can eliminate the need for unnecessary checkups and screening tests in some cases. A positive result can direct a person toward available prevention, monitoring, and treatment options. Some test results can also help people make decisions about having children. Newborn screening can identify genetic disorders early in life so treatment can be started as early as possible.

What Are The Risks And Limitations Of Genetic Testing?

The physical risks associated with most genetic tests are very small, particularly for those tests that require only a blood sample or buccal smear (a procedure that samples cells from the inside surface of the cheek). The procedures used for prenatal testing carry a small but real risk of losing the pregnancy (miscarriage) because they require a sample of amniotic fluid or tissue from around the fetus.

Many of the risks associated with genetic testing involve the emotional, social, or financial consequences of the test results. People may feel angry, depressed, anxious, or guilty about their results. In some cases, genetic testing creates tension within a family because the results can reveal information about other family members in addition to the person who is tested. The possibility of genetic discrimination in employment or insurance is also a concern.

Genetic testing can provide only limited information about an inherited condition. The test often can't determine if a person will show symptoms of a disorder, how severe the symptoms will be, or whether the disorder will progress over time. Another major limitation is the lack of treatment strategies for many genetic disorders once they are diagnosed.

A genetics professional can explain in detail the benefits, risks, and limitations of a particular test. It is important that any person who is considering genetic testing understand and weigh these factors before making a decision.

Chapter 34

Pregnancy Complications

Complications of pregnancy are health problems that occur during pregnancy. They can involve the mother's health, the baby's health, or both. Some women have health problems that arise during pregnancy, and other women have health problems before they become pregnant that could lead to complications. It is very important for women to receive healthcare before and during pregnancy to decrease the risk of pregnancy complications.

Before Pregnancy

Make sure to talk to your doctor about health problems you have now or have had in the past. If you are receiving treatment for a health problem, your healthcare provider might want to change the way your health problem is managed. For example, some medicines used to treat health problems could be harmful if taken during pregnancy. At the same time, stopping medicines that you need could be more harmful than the risks posed should you become pregnant. In addition, be sure to discuss any problems you had in any previous pregnancy. If health problems are under control and you get good prenatal care, you are likely to have a normal, healthy baby.

During Pregnancy

Pregnancy symptoms and complications can range from mild and annoying discomforts to severe, sometimes life-threatening, illnesses. Sometimes it can be difficult for a woman to determine which symptoms are normal and which are not. Problems during pregnancy may

About This Chapter: This chapter includes text excerpted from "Pregnancy Complications," Centers for Disease Control and Prevention (CDC), June 17, 2016.

include physical and mental conditions that affect the health of the mother or the baby. These problems can be caused by or can be made worse by being pregnant. Many problems are mild and do not progress; however, when they do, they may harm the mother or her baby. Keep in mind that there are ways to manage problems that come up during pregnancy. Always contact your prenatal care provider if you have any concerns during your pregnancy.

The following are some common maternal health conditions or problems a woman may experience during pregnancy—

Anemia

Anemia is having lower than the normal number of healthy red blood cells. Treating the underlying cause of the anemia will help restore the number of healthy red blood cells. Women with pregnancy related anemia may feel tired and weak. This can be helped by taking iron and folic acid supplements. Your healthcare provider will check your iron levels throughout pregnancy.

Urinary Tract Infections (UTI)

A UTI is a bacterial infection in the urinary tract. You may have a UTI if you have—

- Pain or burning when you use the bathroom.
- Fever, tiredness, or shakiness.
- An urge to use the bathroom often.
- Pressure in your lower belly.
- Urine that smells bad or looks cloudy or reddish.
- Nausea or back pain.

If you think you have a UTI, it is important to see your healthcare provider. He/she can tell if you have a UTI by testing a sample of your urine. Treatment with antibiotics to kill the infection will make it better, often in one or two days. Some women carry bacteria in their bladder without having symptoms. Your healthcare provider will likely test your urine in early pregnancy to see if this is the case and treat you with antibiotics if necessary.

Mental Health Conditions

Some women experience depression during or after pregnancy. Symptoms of depression are:

- A low or sad mood.

- Loss of interest in fun activities.

- Changes in appetite, sleep, and energy.

- Problems thinking, concentrating, and making decisions.

- Feelings of worthlessness, shame, or guilt.

- Thoughts that life is not worth living.

When many of these symptoms occur together and last for more than a week or two at a time, this is probably depression. Depression that persists during pregnancy can make it hard for a woman to care for herself and her unborn baby. Having depression before pregnancy also is a risk factor for postpartum depression. Getting treatment is important for both mother and baby. If you have a history of depression, it is important to discuss this with your healthcare provider early in pregnancy so that a plan for management can be made.

Hypertension (High Blood Pressure)

Chronic poorly-controlled high blood pressure before and during pregnancy puts a pregnant woman and her baby at risk for problems. It is associated with an increased risk for maternal complications such as preeclampsia, placental abruption (when the placenta separates from the wall of the uterus), and gestational diabetes. These women also face a higher risk for poor birth outcomes such as preterm delivery, having an infant small for his/her gestational age, and infant death. The most important thing to do is to discuss blood pressure problems with your provider before you become pregnant so that appropriate treatment and control of your blood pressure occurs before pregnancy. Getting treatment for high blood pressure is important before, during, and after pregnancy.

Gestational Diabetes Mellitus (GDM)

Gestational Diabetes Mellitus (GDM) is diagnosed during pregnancy and can lead to pregnancy complications. GDM is when the body cannot effectively process sugars and starches (carbohydrates), leading to high sugar levels in the blood stream. Most women with GDM can control their blood sugar levels by a following a healthy meal plan from their healthcare provider and getting regular physical activity. Some women also need insulin to keep blood sugar levels under control. Doing so is important because poorly controlled diabetes increases the risk of—

- Cesarean birth.

- Early delivery.

- Preeclampsia.

- Having a big baby, which can complicate delivery.

- Having a baby born with low blood sugar, breathing problems, and jaundice.

Although GDM usually resolves after pregnancy, women who had GDM have a higher risk of developing diabetes in the future.

Obesity And Weight Gain

Recent studies suggest that the heavier a woman is before she becomes pregnant, the greater her risk of pregnancy complications, including preeclampsia, GDM, stillbirth and Cesarean delivery. Also, Centers for Disease Control and Prevention (CDC) research has shown that obesity during pregnancy is associated with increased use of healthcare and physician services, and longer hospital stays for delivery. Overweight and obese women who lose weight before pregnancy are likely to have healthier pregnancies.

Infections

During pregnancy, your baby is protected from many illnesses, like the common cold or a passing stomach bug. But some infections can be harmful to you, your baby, or both. Easy steps, such as hand washing, and avoiding certain foods, can help protect you from some infections. You won't always know if you have an infection—sometimes you won't even feel sick. If you think you might have an infection or think you are at risk, see your healthcare provider.

Hyperemesis Gravidarum

Many women have some nausea or vomiting, or "morning sickness," particularly during the first 3 months of pregnancy. The cause of nausea and vomiting during pregnancy is believed to be rapidly rising blood levels of a hormone called HCG (human chorionic

---

When To Call The Doctor

Call your doctor or midwife as soon as you can if you:

- Are bleeding or leaking fluid from the vagina
- Are vomiting or have persistent nausea

- Feel discomfort, pain, or burning with urination
- Feel dizzy
- Get severe or long-lasting headaches
- Have a fever or chills
- Have discomfort, pain, or cramping in the lower abdomen
- Have problems seeing or blurred vision
- Have sudden or severe swelling in the face, hands, or fingers
- Have thoughts of harming yourself or your baby
- Suspect your baby is moving less than normal after 28 weeks of pregnancy (If you count less than 10 movements within two hours.)

(Source: "Pregnancy Complications," Office on Women's Health (OWH), U.S. Department of Health and Human Services (HHS).)

gonadotropin), which is released by the placenta. However, hyperemesis gravidarum occurs when there is severe, persistent nausea and vomiting during pregnancy—more extreme than "morning sickness." This can lead to weight loss and dehydration and may require intensive treatment.

Chapter 35
Anemia During Pregnancy

Anemia is a condition in which your blood has a lower than normal number of red blood cells.

Anemia also can occur if your red blood cells don't contain enough hemoglobin. Hemoglobin is an iron-rich protein that gives blood its red color. This protein helps red blood cells carry oxygen from the lungs to the rest of the body.

If you have anemia, your body doesn't get enough oxygen-rich blood. As a result, you may feel tired or weak. You also may have other symptoms, such as shortness of breath, dizziness, or headaches.

(Source: "What Is Anemia?" National Heart, Lung, and Blood Institute (NHLBI).)

What Are The Types And Causes Of Anemia?[1]

Anemia happens when:

1. The body loses too much blood (such as with heavy periods, certain diseases, and trauma); or

2. The body has problems making red blood cells; or

About This Chapter: This chapter includes text excerpted from documents published by three public domain sources. Text under the headings marked 1 are excerpted from "Anemia Fact Sheet," National Women's Health Information Center (NWHIC), Office on Women's Health (OWH), July 16, 2012. Reviewed March 2017; Text under headings marked 2 are excerpted from "The Effect Of Iron Deficiency Anemia During Pregnancy," ClinicalTrials.gov, U.S. National Institutes of Health (NIH), October 27, 2015; Text under the headings marked 3 are excerpted from "Anemia In Pregnancy," National Guideline Clearinghouse (NGC), Agency for Healthcare Research and Quality (AHRQ), 2013. Reviewed March 2017.

3. Red blood cells break down or die faster than the body can replace them with new ones; or

4. More than one of these problems happen at the same time.

There are many types of anemia, all with different causes:

- **Iron deficiency anemia (IDA).** IDA is the most common type of anemia. IDA happens when you don't have enough iron in your body. You need iron to make hemoglobin. People with this type of anemia are sometimes said to have "iron-poor blood" or "tired blood."

A person can have a low iron level because of blood loss. In women, iron and red blood cells are lost when bleeding occurs from very heavy and long periods, as well as from childbirth. Women also can lose iron and red blood cells from uterine fibroids, which can bleed slowly. Other ways iron and red blood cells can be lost include:

- Ulcers, colon polyps, or colon cancer

- Regular use of aspirin and other drugs for pain

- Infections

- Severe injury

- Surgery

Eating foods low in iron also can cause IDA. Meat, poultry, fish, eggs, dairy products, or iron-fortified foods are the best sources of iron found in food. Pregnancy can cause IDA if a woman doesn't consume enough iron for both her and her unborn baby.

Some people have enough iron in their diet, but have problems absorbing it because of diseases, such as Crohn's disease and Celiac disease, or drugs they are taking.

- **Vitamin deficiency anemia (or megaloblastic anemia).** Low levels of vitamin B12 or folate are the most common causes of this type of anemia.

Vitamin B12 deficiency anemia (or pernicious anemia). This type of anemia happens due to a lack of vitamin B12 in the body. Your body needs vitamin B12 to make red blood cells and to keep your nervous system working normally. This type of anemia occurs most often in people whose bodies are not able to absorb vitamin B12 from food because of an autoimmune disorder. It also can happen because of intestinal problems.

You also can get this type of anemia if the foods you eat don't have enough vitamin B12. Vitamin B12 is found in foods that come from animals. Fortified breakfast cereals also have vitamin B12. Folic acid supplements (pills) can treat this type of anemia. But, folic acid cannot treat nerve damage caused by a lack of vitamin B12.

With this type of anemia, your doctor may not realize that you're not getting enough vitamin B12. Not getting enough vitamin B12 can cause numbness in your legs and feet, problems walking, memory loss, and problems seeing. The treatment depends on the cause. But you may need to get vitamin B12 shots or take special vitamin B12 pills.

Folate deficiency anemia. Folate, also called folic acid, is also needed to make red blood cells. This type of anemia can occur if you don't consume enough folate or if you have problems absorbing vitamins. It also may occur during the third trimester of pregnancy, when your body needs extra folate. Folate is a B vitamin found in foods such as leafy green vegetables, fruits, and dried beans and peas. Folic acid is found in fortified breads, pastas, and cereals.

- **Anemias caused by underlying diseases.** Some diseases can hurt the body's ability to make red blood cells. For example, anemia is common in people with kidney disease. Their kidneys can't make enough of the hormones that signal the body to make red blood cells. Plus, iron is lost in dialysis (what some people with kidney disease must have to take out waste from the blood).

- **Anemias caused by inherited blood disease.** If you have a blood disease in your family, you are at greater risk to also have this disease. Here are some types:

Sickle cell anemia. The red blood cells of people with sickle cell disease are hard and have a curved edge. These cells can get stuck in the small blood vessels, blocking the flow of blood to the organs and limbs. The body destroys sickle red cells quickly. But, it can't make new red blood cells fast enough. These factors cause anemia.

Thalassemia. People with thalassemia make less hemoglobin and fewer red blood cells than normal. This leads to mild or severe anemia. One severe form of this condition is Cooley's anemia.

Aplastic anemia. This is a rare blood disorder in which the body stops making enough new blood cells. All blood cells—red cells, white cells, and platelets—are affected. Low levels of red blood cells leads to anemia. With low levels of white blood cells, the body is less able to fight infections. With too few platelets, the blood can't clot normally. This can be caused by many things:

- Cancer treatments (radiation or chemotherapy)

- Exposure to toxic chemicals (like those used in some insecticides, paint, and household cleaners)

215

- Some drugs (like those that treat rheumatoid arthritis)
- Autoimmune diseases (like lupus)
- Viral infections
- Family diseases passed on by genes, such as Fanconi anemia

What Are The Signs Of Anemia?[1]

Anemia takes some time to develop. In the beginning, you may not have any signs or they may be mild. But as it gets worse, you may have these symptoms:

- Fatigue (very common)
- Weakness (very common)
- Dizziness
- Headache
- Numbness or coldness in your hands and feet
- Low body temperature
- Pale skin
- Rapid or irregular heartbeat
- Shortness of breath
- Chest pain
- Irritability
- Not doing well at work or in school

All of these signs and symptoms can occur because your heart has to work harder to pump more oxygen-rich blood through the body.

Iron Deficiency Anemia[2]

Iron deficiency anemia during pregnancy is a significant worldwide health problem, affecting 22 percent of pregnant women in industrialized countries and 52 percent in non-industrialized countries. Iron deficiency anemia during pregnancy is associated with increased maternal as well as fetal morbidity, including prematurity, low birth-weight and perinatal and infant loss. Therefore, routine iron supplementation during the second half of pregnancy has been recommended once daily. Others, however, support a selective iron supplementation only for women with iron deficiency anemia, in order to avoid the increased risk of haemoconcentration associated with routine iron supplementation. Unfortunately, compliance to either iron-supplementation programs, especially among pregnant women, is poor, due in part to the side effects associated with these preparations.

Effects Of Iron Deficiency Anemia During Pregnancy[3]

- Iron deficiency anemia during pregnancy has been associated with an increased risk of low birth weight, preterm delivery, and perinatal mortality.

- Severe anemia with maternal hemoglobin (Hgb) levels less than 6 g/dL has been associated with abnormal fetal oxygenation resulting in nonreassuring fetal heart rate patterns, reduced amniotic fluid volume, fetal cerebral vasodilatation, and fetal death. Thus, maternal transfusion should be considered for fetal indications.

- Iron supplementation decreases the prevalence of maternal anemia at delivery.

How Much Iron Do I Need If I Am Pregnant?[1]

Pregnant women need to consume twice as much iron as women who are not pregnant. But about half of all pregnant women do not get enough iron. During pregnancy, your body needs more iron because of the growing fetus, the higher volume of blood, and blood loss during delivery. If a pregnant woman does not get enough iron for herself or her growing baby, she has an increased chance of having preterm birth and a low-birth-weight baby. If you're pregnant, follow these tips:

- Make sure you get 27mg of iron every day. Take an iron supplement (pill). It may be part of your prenatal vitamin. Start taking it at your first prenatal visit.

- Get tested for anemia at your first prenatal visit.

- Ask if you need to be tested for anemia 4 to 6 weeks after delivery.

Treatment[2]

Currently, there are many iron preparations available containing different types of iron salts, including ferrous sulfate, ferrous fumarate, ferrous ascorbate but common adverse drug reactions found with these preparations are mainly gastrointestinal intolerance like nausea, vomiting, constipation, diarrhea, abdominal pain, while ferrous bis-glycinate rarely make complication.

Product resulting from the reaction of a metal ion from a soluble salt with amino acids to form coordinate covalent bonds, the resulting molecule is called as chelate and chemical bonding process is called chelation. Ferrous bis-glycinate is highly stable and totally nutritionally functional chelate it is an amino acid fully reacted chelate which is formed by the binding of two molecules of glycine to one Fe^{2+} atom.

Does Birth Control Affect My Risk For Anemia?[1]

It could. Some women who take birth control pills have less bleeding during their periods. This would lower their risk for anemia. But women who use an intrauterine device (IUD) may have more bleeding and increase their chances of getting anemia. Talk to your doctor.

I Am A Vegetarian. What Steps Should I Take To Make Sure I Get Enough Iron?[1]

It depends on the food choices you make. Since meat, poultry, and seafood are the best sources of iron found in food, some vegetarians may need to take a higher amount of iron each day than what is recommended for other people. Follow the tips above to prevent anemia, and try to take vitamin C with the iron-rich foods you eat.

Recommendations[3]

All pregnant women should be screened for anemia, and those with iron deficiency anemia should be treated with supplemental iron, in addition to prenatal vitamins.

Patients with anemia other than iron deficiency anemia should be further evaluated.

Failure to respond to iron therapy should prompt further investigation and may suggest an incorrect diagnosis, coexisting disease, malabsorption (sometimes caused by the use of enteric-coated tablets or concomitant use of antacids), noncompliance, or blood loss.

- Interventions and Practices Considered

- Iron supplementation

- Screening for anemia during pregnancy

- Maternal transfusion in case of severe anemia
- Parenteral iron for patients who cannot tolerate oral iron: iron dextran or ferrous sucrose
- Autologous transfusion
- Prenatal vitamin supplementation

Chapter 36

Preeclampsia And Eclampsia

What Are Preeclampsia And Eclampsia?

Preeclampsia and eclampsia are part of the spectrum of high blood pressure, or hypertensive, disorders that can occur during pregnancy. At the mild end of the spectrum is **gestational hypertension,** which occurs when a woman who previously had normal blood pressure develops high blood pressure when she is more than 20 weeks pregnant. This problem occurs without other symptoms. Typically, gestational hypertension does not harm the mother or fetus and resolves after delivery. However, about 15–25 percent of women with gestational hypertension will go on to develop preeclampsia.

Preeclampsia is a condition that develops in women with previously normal blood pressure at 20 weeks of pregnancy or greater and includes increased blood pressure (levels greater than 140/90), increased swelling, and protein in the urine. The condition can be serious, and, if it is severe enough to affect brain function, causing seizures or coma, it is called **eclampsia.**

One of the serious complications of hypertensive disorders in pregnancy is **HELLP syndrome,** when a pregnant woman with preeclampsia or eclampsia sustains damage to the liver and blood cells. The letters in the name HELLP stand for the following problems:

- **H** – **H**emolysis, in which oxygen-carrying red blood cells break down

- **EL** – **E**levated **L**iver enzymes, showing damage to the liver

- **LP** – **L**ow **P**latelet count, in which the cells responsible for stopping bleeding are low

---

About This Chapter: This chapter includes text excerpted from "Preeclampsia And Eclampsia: Condition Information," *Eunice Kennedy Shriver* National Institute of Child Health and Human Development (NICHD), December 3, 2012. Reviewed March 2017.

What Causes Preeclampsia And Eclampsia?

The causes of preeclampsia and eclampsia are not known. These disorders previously were believed to be caused by a toxin in the blood (referred to as toxemia), but healthcare providers now know that is not true.

To learn more about preeclampsia and eclampsia, scientists are investigating many factors that could contribute to the development and progression of these diseases, including:

- Cardiovascular and inflammatory changes

- Environmental exposures

- Genetic factors

- Hormonal imbalances

- Maternal immunology and autoimmune disorders

- Nutritional factors

- Placental abnormalities, such as insufficient blood flow

What Are The Risks Of Preeclampsia And Eclampsia To The Mother?

Risks During Pregnancy

Preeclampsia during pregnancy is mild in 75 percent of cases. However, a woman can progress from mild to severe preeclampsia or full eclampsia very quickly—even in a matter of days—especially if she is not treated. Both preeclampsia and eclampsia can cause serious health problems for the mother and infant.

Preeclampsia affects the placenta as well as the mother's kidneys, liver, brain, and other organ and blood systems. The condition could lead to a separation of the placenta from the uterus (referred to as placental abruption), preterm delivery, and pregnancy loss. In some cases, preeclampsia can lead to organ failure or stroke. In severe cases, preeclampsia can develop into eclampsia, which can lead to seizures. Seizures in eclampsia cause a woman to lose consciousness, fall to the ground, and twitch uncontrollably. If not treated, these conditions can cause the death of the mother and/or the fetus.

Expecting mothers rarely die from preeclampsia in the developed world, but it is still a major cause of illness and death globally. According to the World Health Organization

(WHO), preeclampsia and eclampsia cause 14 percent of maternal deaths each year, or about 50,000 to 75,000 women worldwide.

Risks After Pregnancy

In uncomplicated preeclampsia, the mother's high blood pressure and increased protein in the urine usually resolve within 6 weeks of the infant's birth. Studies, however, have shown that women who have had preeclampsia are four times more likely to develop hypertension and twice as likely to develop ischemic heart disease (reduced blood supply to the heart muscle, which can cause heart attacks), a blood clot in a vein, and stroke.

Less commonly, mothers who had preeclampsia during pregnancy could experience permanent damage to their organs. Preeclampsia could lead to kidney and liver damage or fluid in the lungs.

What Are The Risks Of Preeclampsia And Eclampsia To The Fetus?

Preeclampsia affects the flow of blood to the placenta. Risks to the fetus include:

- Lack of oxygen and nutrients, leading to poor fetal growth due to preeclampsia itself or if the placenta separates from the uterus before birth (placental abruption)

- Preterm birth

- Stillbirth if placental abruption leads to heavy bleeding in the mother

Stillbirths are more likely to occur when the mother has a more severe form of preeclampsia, including HELLP syndrome.

Preeclampsia also can raise the risk of some long-term health issues related to preterm birth, including learning disorders, cerebral palsy, epilepsy, deafness, and blindness. Infants born preterm also risk extended hospitalization and small size. Infants who experienced poor growth in the uterus may later be at higher risk of diabetes, congestive heart failure, and hypertension.

How Many Women Are Affected By Or At Risk Of Preeclampsia?

The exact number of women who develop preeclampsia is not known. Some scientists and healthcare providers estimate that preeclampsia affects 5–10 percent of all pregnancies globally. The rates are lower in the United States (about 3–5 percent of women), but it is estimated to account for 40–60 percent of maternal deaths in developing countries. Disorders related to high blood pressure are the second leading cause of stillbirths and early neonatal deaths in developing nations.

In addition, HELLP syndrome occurs in about 10–20 percent of all women with severe preeclampsia or eclampsia.

Risk Factors For Preeclampsia

Preeclampsia occurs primarily in first pregnancies. Other factors that can increase a woman's risk include:

- Chronic high blood pressure or kidney disease before pregnancy

- High blood pressure or preeclampsia in an earlier pregnancy

- Obesity

- Women who are younger than age 20 or older than 35

- Women who are pregnant with more than one fetus

- Being African American

- Having a family history of preeclampsia

According to the World Health Organization, among women who have had preeclampsia, about 20–40 percent of their daughters and 11–37 percent of their sisters also will get the disorder.

Preeclampsia is more common among women who have histories of certain health conditions, such as migraine headaches, diabetes, rheumatoid arthritis, lupus, scleroderma, urinary tract infection, gum disease, polycystic ovary syndrome, multiple sclerosis, gestational diabetes, and sickle cell disease.

Preeclampsia is also more common in pregnancies resulting from egg donation, donor insemination, or in vitro fertilization.

What Are The Symptoms Of Preeclampsia, Eclampsia, And HELLP Syndrome?

Preeclampsia

Possible symptoms of preeclampsia include:

- High blood pressure

- Too much protein in the urine
- Swelling in a woman's face and hands (a woman's feet might swell too, but swollen feet are common during pregnancy and may not signal a problem)
- Systemic problems, such as headache, blurred vision, and right upper quadrant abdominal pain

Eclampsia

Women with preeclampsia can develop seizures. The following symptoms are cause for immediate concern:

- Severe headache
- Vision problems, such as temporary blindness
- Abdominal pain, especially in the upper right area of the belly
- Nausea and vomiting
- Smaller urine output or not urinating very often

HELLP Syndrome

HELLP syndrome can lead to serious complications, including liver failure and death.

A pregnant woman with HELLP syndrome might bleed or bruise easily and/or experience abdominal pain, nausea or vomiting, headache, or extreme fatigue. Although most women who develop HELLP syndrome already have high blood pressure and preeclampsia, sometimes the syndrome is the first sign. In addition, HELLP syndrome can occur without a woman having either high blood pressure or protein in her urine.

How Do Healthcare Providers Diagnose Preeclampsia, Eclampsia, And HELLP Syndrome?

A healthcare provider should check a pregnant woman's blood pressure and urine during each prenatal visit. If the blood pressure reading is considered high (140/90 or higher), especially after the 20th week of pregnancy, the healthcare provider will likely perform more extensive lab tests to look for extra protein in the urine (called proteinuria) as well as other abnormalities.

Gestational hypertension is diagnosed if the woman has high blood pressure but no protein in the urine. Gestational hypertension occurs when women with normal blood pressure levels before pregnancy develop high blood pressure after 20 weeks of pregnancy. Gestational hypertension can develop into preeclampsia.

Mild preeclampsia is diagnosed when a pregnant woman has:

- Systolic blood pressure (top number) of 140 mmHg or higher or diastolic blood pressure (bottom number) of 90 mmHg or higher

- Urine with 0.3 or more grams of protein in a 24-hour specimen (a collection of every drop of urine within 24 hours)

Severe preeclampsia occurs when a pregnant woman has:

- Systolic blood pressure of 160 mmHg or higher or diastolic blood pressure of 110 mmHg or higher on two occasions at least 6 hours apart

- Urine with 5 or more grams of protein in a 24-hour specimen or 3 or more grams of protein on 2 random urine samples collected at least 4 hours apart

- Test results suggesting blood or liver damage—for example, blood tests that reveal low numbers of red blood cells, low numbers of platelets, or high liver enzymes

- Symptoms that include severe weight gain, difficulty breathing, or fluid buildup

Eclampsia occurs when women with preeclampsia develop seizures.

A healthcare provider may do other tests to assess the health of the mother and fetus, including:

- Blood tests to see how well the mother's liver and kidneys are working

- Blood tests to check blood platelet levels to see how well the mother's blood is clotting

- Blood tests to count the total number of red blood cells in the mother's blood

- A maternal weight check

- An ultrasound to assess the fetus's size

- A check of the fetus's heart rate

- A physical exam to look for swelling in the mother's face, hands, or legs as well as abdominal tenderness or an enlarged liver

HELLP syndrome is diagnosed when laboratory tests show hemolysis, elevated liver enzymes, and low platelets. There also may or may not be extra protein in the urine.

What Are The Treatments For Preeclampsia, Eclampsia, And HELLP Syndrome?

Preeclampsia

The only cure for preeclampsia when it occurs during pregnancy is delivering the fetus. Treatment decisions need to take into account the severity of the condition and the potential for maternal complications, how far along the pregnancy is, and the potential risks to the fetus. Ideally, the healthcare provider will minimize risks to the mother while giving the fetus as much time as possible to mature before delivery.

If the fetus is at 37 weeks or later, the healthcare provider will usually want to deliver it to avoid further complications.

If the fetus is younger than 37 weeks, however, the woman and her healthcare provider may want to consider other options that give the fetus more time to develop, depending on how severe the condition is. A healthcare provider may consider the following treatment options:

- If the preeclampsia is mild, it may be possible to wait to deliver the infant. To help prevent further complications, the healthcare provider may ask the woman to go on bed rest (to try to lower blood pressure and increase the blood flow to the placenta).

- Close monitoring of the woman and her fetus will be needed. Tests for the mother might include blood and urine tests to see if the preeclampsia is progressing (such as tests to assess platelet counts, liver enzymes, kidney function, and urinary protein levels). Tests for the fetus might include ultrasound, heart rate monitoring, assessment of fetal growth, and amniotic fluid assessment.

- Anticonvulsive medication, such as magnesium sulfate, might be used to prevent a seizure.

- In some cases, such as with severe preeclampsia, the woman will be admitted to the hospital so she can be monitored closely. Treatment in the hospital might include intravenous medication to control blood pressure and prevent seizures or other complications as well as steroid injections to help speed up the development of the fetus's lungs.

When a woman has severe preeclampsia, the doctor will probably want to deliver the fetus as soon as possible. Delivery usually is suggested if the pregnancy has lasted more than 34 weeks. If the fetus is less than 34 weeks, the doctor will probably prescribe corticosteroids to help speed up the maturation of the lungs.

In some cases, the doctor must deliver the fetus prematurely, even if that means likely complications for the infant because of the risk of severe maternal complications. The symptoms of preeclampsia usually go away within 6 weeks of delivery.

Eclampsia

Eclampsia—the onset of seizures in a woman with preeclampsia—is considered a medical emergency. Immediate treatment, usually in a hospital, is needed to stop the mother's seizures; treat blood pressure levels that are too high; and deliver the infant.

Magnesium sulfate (a type of mineral) may be given to treat active seizures and prevent future seizures. Antihypertensive medications may be given to lower the blood pressure.

The only cure for gestational eclampsia is to deliver the fetus.

HELLP Syndrome

HELLP syndrome, a special type of severe preeclampsia, can lead to serious complications for the mother, including liver failure and death, as well as the fetus. The healthcare provider may consider the following treatments after a diagnosis of HELLP syndrome:

- Delivery, particularly if the pregnancy is 34 weeks or later.

- Hospitalization to provide intravenous medication to control blood pressure and prevent seizures or other complications as well as steroid injections to help speed up the development of the fetus's lungs.

Chapter 37

Preterm Labor And Birth

What Is Preterm Labor And Birth?

In general, a normal human pregnancy is about 40 weeks long (9.2 months). Healthcare providers now define "full-term" birth as birth that occurs between 39 weeks and 40 weeks and 6 days of pregnancy. Infants born during this time are considered full-term infants.

Infants born in the 37th and 38th weeks of pregnancy—previously called term but now referred to as "early term"—face more health risks than do those born at 39 or 40 weeks.

Deliveries before 37 weeks of pregnancy are considered "preterm" or premature:

- Labor that begins before 37 weeks of pregnancy is preterm or premature labor.

- A birth that occurs before 37 weeks of pregnancy is a preterm or premature birth.

- An infant born before 37 weeks in the womb is a preterm or premature infant. (These infants are commonly called "preemies" as a reference to being born prematurely.)

"Late preterm" refers to 34 weeks through 36 weeks of pregnancy. Infants born during this time are considered late-preterm infants, but they face many of the same health challenges as preterm infants. More than 70 percent of preterm infants are born during the late-preterm time frame.

Preterm birth is the most common cause of infant death and is the leading cause of long-term disability in children. Many organs, including the brain, lungs, and liver, are still developing in the final weeks of pregnancy. The earlier the delivery, the higher the risk of serious disability or death.

About This Chapter: This chapter includes text excerpted from "Preterm Labor And Birth: Condition Information," *Eunice Kennedy Shriver* National Institute of Child Health and Human Development (NICHD), March 16, 2014.

Infants born prematurely are at risk for cerebral palsy (a group of nervous system disorders that affect control of movement and posture and limit activity), developmental delays, and vision and hearing problems.

Late-preterm infants typically have better health outcomes than those born earlier, but they are still three times more likely to die in the first year of life than are full-term infants. Preterm births can also take a heavy emotional and economic toll on families.

What Are The Symptoms Of Preterm Labor?

Preterm labor is any labor that occurs from 20 weeks through 36 weeks of pregnancy. Here are the symptoms:

- Contractions (tightening of stomach muscles, or birth pains) every 10 minutes or more often

- Change in vaginal discharge (leaking fluid or bleeding from the vagina)

- Feeling of pressure in the pelvis (hip) area

- Low, dull backache

- Cramps that feel like menstrual cramps

- Abdominal cramps with or without diarrhea

It is normal for pregnant women to have some uterine contractions throughout the day. It is not normal to have frequent uterine contractions, such as six or more in one hour. Frequent uterine contractions, or tightenings, may cause the cervix to begin to open.

If a woman thinks that she might be having preterm labor, she should call her doctor or go to the hospital to be evaluated.

How Many People Are Affected By Preterm Labor And Birth?

Going into preterm labor does not always mean that a pregnant woman will deliver the baby prematurely. Up to one-half of women who experience preterm labor eventually deliver at 37 weeks of pregnancy or later.

In some cases, intervention from a healthcare provider is needed to stop preterm labor. In other cases, the labor may stop on its own. A woman who thinks she is experiencing preterm labor should contact a healthcare provider immediately.

In 2015, about 1 out of 10 babies was born too early in the United States.

Preterm birth rates decreased from 2007 to 2014 and CDC research shows the decline in preterm births is partly due to fewer teens and young women becoming pregnant.

(Source: "Premature Birth," Centers for Disease Control and Prevention (CDC).)

How Many Women Are At Risk For Preterm Labor And Delivery?

Any pregnant woman could experience preterm labor and delivery. But there are some factors that increase a woman's risk of going into labor or giving birth prematurely.

What Causes Preterm Labor And Birth?

The causes of preterm labor and premature birth are numerous, complex, and only partly understood. Medical, psychosocial, and biological factors may all play a role in preterm labor and birth.

There are three main situations in which preterm labor and premature birth may occur:

- **Spontaneous preterm labor and birth.** This term refers to unintentional, unplanned delivery before the 37th week of pregnancy. This type of preterm birth can result from a number of causes, such as infection or inflammation, although the cause of spontaneous preterm labor and delivery is usually not known. A history of delivering preterm is one of the strongest predictors for subsequent preterm births.

- **Medically indicated preterm birth.** If a serious medical condition—such as preeclampsia—exists, the healthcare provider might recommend a preterm delivery. In these cases, healthcare providers often take steps to keep the baby in the womb as long as possible to allow for additional growth and development, while also monitoring the mother and fetus for health issues. Providers also use additional interventions, such as steroids, to help improve outcomes for the baby.

- **Non-medically indicated (elective) preterm delivery.** Some late-preterm births result from inducing labor or having a Cesarean delivery even though there is not a medical reason to do so, even though this practice is not recommended. Research indicates that even babies born at 37 or 38 weeks of pregnancy are at higher risk for poor health outcomes than are babies born at 39 weeks of pregnancy or later. Therefore, unless there are medical problems, healthcare providers should wait until at least 39 weeks of pregnancy to induce labor or perform a Cesarean delivery to prevent possible health problems.

What Are The Risk Factors For Preterm Labor And Birth?

There are several risk factors for preterm labor and premature birth, including ones that researchers have not yet identified. Some of these risk factors are "modifiable," meaning they can be changed to help reduce the risk. Other factors cannot be changed.

Healthcare providers consider the following factors to put women at high risk for preterm labor or birth:

- Women who have delivered preterm before, or who have experienced preterm labor before, are considered to be at high risk for preterm labor and birth.

- Being pregnant with twins, triplets, or more (called "multiple gestations") or the use of assisted reproductive technology is associated with a higher risk of preterm labor and birth. One study showed that more than 50 percent of twin births occurred preterm, compared with only 10 percent of births of single infants.

- Women with certain abnormalities of the reproductive organs are at greater risk for preterm labor and birth than are women who do not have these abnormalities. For instance, women who have a short cervix (the lower part of the uterus) or whose cervix shortens in the second trimester (fourth through sixth months) of pregnancy instead of the third trimester are at high risk for preterm delivery.

Certain medical conditions, including some that occur only during pregnancy, also place a woman at higher risk for preterm labor and delivery. Some of these conditions include:

- Urinary tract infections

- Sexually transmitted infections

- Certain vaginal infections, such as bacterial vaginosis and trichomoniasis

- High blood pressure

- Bleeding from the vagina

- Certain developmental abnormalities in the fetus

- Pregnancy resulting from in vitro fertilization

- Being underweight or obese before pregnancy

- Short time period between pregnancies (less than 6 months between a birth and the beginning of the next pregnancy)

- Placenta previa, a condition in which the placenta grows in the lowest part of the uterus and covers all or part of the opening to the cervix

- Being at risk for rupture of the uterus (when the wall of the uterus rips open). Rupture of the uterus is more likely if you have had a prior Cesarean delivery or have had a uterine fibroid removed.

- Diabetes (high blood sugar) and gestational diabetes (which occurs only during pregnancy)

- Blood clotting problems

Other factors that may increase risk for preterm labor and premature birth include:

- Ethnicity. Preterm labor and birth occur more often among certain racial and ethnic groups. Infants of African American mothers are 50 percent more likely to be born preterm than are infants of white mothers.

> In 2015, the rate of preterm birth among African-American women (13%) was about 50 percent higher than the rate of preterm birth among white women (9%).
>
> *(Source: "Premature Birth," Centers for Disease Control and Prevention (CDC).)*

- Age of the mother.
  - Women younger than age 18 are more likely to have a preterm delivery.
  - Women older than age 35 are also at risk of having preterm infants because they are more likely to have other conditions (such as high blood pressure and diabetes) that can cause complications requiring preterm delivery.

- Certain lifestyle and environmental factors, including:
  - Late or no healthcare during pregnancy
  - Smoking
  - Drinking alcohol
  - Using illegal drugs
  - Domestic violence, including physical, sexual, or emotional abuse
  - Lack of social support

- Stress

- Long working hours with long periods of standing

- Exposure to certain environmental pollutants

Is It Possible To Predict Which Women Are More Likely To Have Preterm Labor And Birth?

Currently, there is no definitive way to predict preterm labor or premature birth. Many research studies are focusing on this important issue. By identifying which women are at increased risk, healthcare providers may be able to provide early interventions, treatments, and close monitoring of these pregnancies to prevent preterm delivery or to improve health outcomes.

However, in some situations, healthcare providers know that a preterm delivery is very likely. Some of these situations are described below.

Shortened Cervix

As a preparation for birth, the cervix (the lower part of the uterus) naturally shortens late in pregnancy. However, in some women, the cervix shortens prematurely, around the fourth or fifth month of pregnancy, increasing the risk for preterm delivery.

In some cases, a healthcare provider may recommend measuring a pregnant woman's cervical length, especially if she previously had preterm labor or a preterm birth. Ultrasound scans may be used to measure cervical length and identify women with a shortened cervix.

"Incompetent" Cervix

The cervix normally remains closed during pregnancy. In some cases, the cervix starts to open early, before a fetus is ready to be born. Healthcare providers may refer to a cervix that begins to open as an "incompetent" cervix. The process of cervical opening is painless and unnoticeable, without labor contractions or cramping.

Approximately 5 to 10 out of 1,000 pregnant women are diagnosed as having an incompetent cervix.

To try to prevent preterm birth, a doctor may place a stitch around the cervix to keep it closed. This procedure is called cervical cerclage. NICHD-supported research has found that, in women with a prior preterm birth who have a short cervix, cerclage may improve the likelihood of a full-term delivery.

How Do Healthcare Providers Diagnose Preterm Labor?

If a woman is concerned that she could be showing signs of preterm labor, she should call her healthcare provider or go to the hospital to be evaluated. In particular, a woman should call if she has more than six contractions in an hour or if fluid or blood is leaking from the vagina.

Physical Exam

If a woman is experiencing signs of labor, the healthcare provider may perform a pelvic exam to see if:

- The membranes have ruptured

- The cervix is beginning to get thinner (efface)

- The cervix is beginning to open (dilate)

Any of these situations could mean the woman is in preterm labor.

Providers may also do an ultrasound exam and use a monitor to electronically record contractions and the fetal heart rate.

Fetal Fibronectin (fFN) Test

This test is used to detect whether the protein fetal fibronectin is being produced. fFN is like a biological "glue" between the uterine lining and the membrane that surrounds the fetus.

Normally fFN is detectable in the pregnant woman's secretions from the vagina and cervix early in the pregnancy (up to 22 weeks, or about 5 months) and again toward the end of the pregnancy (1 to 3 weeks before labor begins). It is usually not present between 24 and 34 weeks of pregnancy (5½ to 8½ months). If fFN is detected during this time, it may be a sign that the woman may be at risk of preterm labor and birth.

In most cases, the fFN test is performed on women who are showing signs of preterm labor. Testing for fFN can predict with about 50 percent accuracy which pregnant women showing signs of preterm labor are likely to have a preterm delivery. It is typically used for its negative predictive value, meaning that if it is negative, it is unlikely that a woman will deliver within the next 7 days.

What Treatments Are Used To Prevent Preterm Labor And Birth?

Currently, treatment options for preventing preterm labor or birth are somewhat limited, in part because the cause of preterm labor or birth is often unknown. But there are a few options, described below.

Hormone treatment. The only preventive drug therapy is progesterone, a hormone produced by the body during pregnancy, which is given to women at risk of preterm birth, such as those with a prior preterm birth. The NICHD's Maternal-Fetal Medicine Units (MFMU) Network found that progesterone given to women at risk of preterm birth due to a prior preterm birth reduces chances of a subsequent preterm birth by one-third. This preventive therapy is given beginning at 16 weeks of gestation and continues to 37 weeks of gestation. The treatment works among all ethnic groups and can improve outcomes for infants.

Cerclage. A surgical procedure called cervical cerclage is sometimes used to try to prevent early labor in women who have an incompetent (weak) cervix and have experienced early pregnancy loss accompanied by a painless opening (dilation) of the cervix (the bottom part of the uterus). In the cerclage procedure, a doctor stitches the cervix closed. The stitch is then removed closer to the woman's due date.

Bed rest. Contrary to expectations, confining the mother to bed rest does not help to prevent preterm birth. In fact, bed rest can make preterm birth even more likely among some women.

Women should discuss all of their treatment options—including the risks and benefits—with their healthcare providers. If possible, these discussions should occur during regular prenatal care visits, before there is any urgency, to allow for a complete discussion of all the issues.

What Treatments Can Reduce The Chances Of Preterm Labor And Birth?

If a pregnant woman is showing signs of preterm labor, her doctor will often try treatments to stop labor and prolong the pregnancy until the fetus is more fully developed. Treatments include therapies to try to stop labor (tocolytics) and medications administered before birth to improve outcomes for the infant if born preterm (antenatal steroids to improve the respiratory outcomes and neuroprotective medications such as magnesium sulfate).

Medications To Delay Labor

Drugs called tocolytics can be given to many women with symptoms of preterm labor. These drugs can slow or stop contractions of the uterus and may prevent labor for 2 to 7 days. One common treatment for delaying labor is magnesium sulfate, given to the pregnant woman intravenously through a needle inserted in an arm vein.

Medications To Speed Development Of The Fetus

Tocolytics may provide the extra time for treatment with corticosteroids to speed up development of the fetus's lungs and some other organs or for the pregnant woman to get to a hospital that offers specialized care for preterm infants. Corticosteroids can be particularly effective if the pregnancy is between 24 and 34 weeks (between 5½ and 7¾ months) and the woman's healthcare provider suspects that the birth may occur within the next week. Intravenously delivered magnesium sulfate may also reduce the risk of cerebral palsy if the child is born early.

What Methods Do Not Work To Prevent Preterm Labor?

Researchers have found that some methods for trying to stop preterm labor are not as effective as once thought. These include:

- Home uterine monitors

- Routine screening of all asymptomatic women for bacterial vaginosis (*Trichomonas vaginalis*) infection. Routine screening and treatment with antibiotics did not reduce preterm birth; in fact, the latter increased the risk of preterm birth.

Chapter 38
Asthma Medication And Pregnancy

Asthma is a chronic (long-term) lung disease that inflames and narrows the airways. Asthma causes recurring periods of wheezing (a whistling sound when you breathe), chest tightness, shortness of breath, and coughing. The coughing often occurs at night or early in the morning.

(Source: "What Is Asthma?" National Heart, Lung, and Blood Institute (NHLBI).)

Maternal Asthma Medication Use And The Risk Of Selected Birth Defects

Researchers used data from the National Birth Defects Prevention Study (NBDPS) to examine maternal asthma medication use during pregnancy and the risk of certain birth defects.

Asthma—A Disease That Affects The Lungs

Asthma is a common disease during pregnancy, affecting about 4–12 percent of pregnant women. About 3 percent of pregnant women use asthma medications, including bronchodilators or anti-inflammatory drugs. Guidelines recommend that women with asthma continue to use medication to control their condition during pregnancy. However, the safety data on using asthma medications during pregnancy are limited.

About This Chapter: Text under the heading "Maternal Asthma Medication Use And The Risk Of Selected Birth Defects" is excerpted from "Key Findings: Maternal Asthma Medication Use And The Risk Of Selected Birth Defects," Centers for Disease Control and Prevention (CDC), October 22, 2014; Text under the heading "Asthma Medicine And Pregnancy" is excerpted from "Medicine And Pregnancy," U.S. Food and Drug Administration (FDA), January 10, 2017.

Main Findings From This Study

- Data from the study showed that using asthma medication during pregnancy
  - Did not increase the risk for most of the birth defects studied.
  - Might increase the risk for some birth defects, such as esophageal atresia (birth defect of the esophagus or food tube), anorectal atresia (birth defect of the anus), and omphalocele (birth defect of the abdominal wall).
- The most commonly reported asthma medications used during pregnancy were
  - Albuterol (2–3 percent of women)
  - Fluticasone (About 1 percent of women)
- It was difficult to determine if asthma or other health problems related to having asthma increased the risk for these birth defects, or if the increased risk was from the medication use during pregnancy.

Medication During Pregnancy: CDC Activities

About 1 in every 33 babies is born with a birth defect. Birth defects are one of the leading causes of infant deaths, accounting for more than 20 percent of all infant deaths. Centers for Disease Control and Prevention (CDC) is committed to working with its partners and the public to build a comprehensive approach to understanding and communicating the risks of birth defects that potentially are associated with the use of medications during pregnancy.

- Research: CDC funds a large study of birth defects called the National Birth Defects Prevention Study. This study is working to identify risk factors for birth defects and to answer questions about some medications taken during pregnancy.
- Technical expertise: CDC works with staff from the U.S. Food and Drug Administration (FDA) and other professionals to help conduct studies on the effects of medication use during pregnancy and ways to prevent harmful effects.

Asthma Medicine And Pregnancy

Are you pregnant and taking medicines? You are not alone. Many women need to take medicines when they are pregnant. There are about six million pregnancies in the United States. each year, and 50 percent of pregnant women say that they take at least one medicine.

Some women take medicines for health problems, like diabetes, morning sickness or high blood pressure that can start or get worse when a woman is pregnant. Others take medicines before they realize they are pregnant.

Accidental Exposure

Sometimes women take medication before they realize that they are pregnant. When this happens, they may worry about the effects of the medication on their unborn baby. The first thing a woman who is pregnant or who is planning on becoming pregnant should do is talk with her healthcare provider. Some medications are harmful when taken during pregnancy, but others are unlikely to cause harm.

(Source: "Medications And Pregnancy," Centers for Disease Control and Prevention (CDC).)

Pregnancy can be an exciting time. However, this time can also make you feel uneasy if you are not sure how your medicines will affect your baby. Not all medicines are safe to take when you are pregnant. Even headache or pain medicine may not be safe during certain times in your pregnancy.

1. Ask Questions

Always talk to your healthcare provider before you take any medicines, herbs, or vitamins. Don't stop taking your medicines until your healthcare provider says that it is OK.

Use these questions to help you talk to your doctor, nurse, or pharmacist:

- **Will I need to change my medicines if I want to get pregnant?** Before you get pregnant, work with your healthcare provider to make a plan to help you safely use your medicines.

- **How might this medicine affect my baby?** Ask about the benefits and risks for you and your baby.

- **What medicines and herbs should I avoid?** Some drugs can harm your baby during different stages of your pregnancy. At these times, your healthcare provider may have you take something else.

- **Will I need to take more or less of my medicine?** Your heart and kidneys work harder when you are pregnant. This makes medicines pass through your body faster than usual.

- **Can I keep taking this medicine when I start breastfeeding?** Some drugs can get into your breast milk and affect your baby.

- **What kind of vitamins should I take?** Ask about special vitamins for pregnant women called pre-natal vitamins.

Pre-Natal Vitamins

Some dietary supplements may have too much or too little of the vitamins that you need. Talk to your healthcare provider about what kind of pre-natal vitamins you should take.

What is folic acid? Folic acid helps to prevent birth defects of the baby's brain or spine. Ask about how much folic acid you should take before you become pregnant and through the first part of your pregnancy.

---

2. Read The Label

Check the drug label and other information you get with your medicine to learn about the possible risks for women who are pregnant or breastfeeding. The labeling tells you what is known about how the drugs might affect pregnant women. Your healthcare provider can help you decide if you should take the medicine.

New Prescription Drug Information

The prescription drug labels are changing. The new labels will replace the old A, B, C, D and X categories with more helpful information about a medicine's risks. The labels will also have more information on whether the medicine gets into breast milk and how it can possibly affect the baby.

3. Be Smart Online

Ask your doctor, nurse, or pharmacist about the information you get online. Some websites say that drugs are safe to take during pregnancy, but you should check with your healthcare provider first. Every woman's body is different. It may not be safe for you.

- Do not trust that a product is safe just because it says 'natural'. Check with your health-care provider before you use a product that you heard about in a chat room or group.

4. Report Problems

First, tell your healthcare provider about any problems you have with your medicine. Also, tell FDA about any serious problems you have after taking a medicine.

- Call 800-FDA-1088 (800-332-1088) to get a reporting form sent to you by mail.

- Report problems online.

What To Report To FDA

You should report problems like serious side effects, product quality problems and product use errors. Report problems with these products:

- human drugs

- medical devices

- blood products and other biologics (except vaccines)

- medical foods

Chapter 39

If You Are Pregnant And Have Diabetes

If you have diabetes and plan to have a baby, you should try to get your blood glucose levels close to your target range before you get pregnant.

Staying in your target range during pregnancy, which may be different than when you aren't pregnant, is also important. High blood glucose, also called blood sugar, can harm your baby during the first weeks of pregnancy, even before you know you are pregnant. If you have diabetes and are already pregnant, see your doctor as soon as possible to make a plan to manage your diabetes. Working with your healthcare team and following your diabetes management plan can help you have a healthy pregnancy and a healthy baby.

If you develop diabetes for the first time while you are pregnant, you have gestational diabetes.

How Can Diabetes Affect My Baby?

A baby's organs, such as the brain, heart, kidneys, and lungs, start forming during the first 8 weeks of pregnancy. High blood glucose levels can be harmful during this early stage and can increase the chance that your baby will have birth defects, such as heart defects or defects of the brain or spine.

High blood glucose levels during pregnancy can also increase the chance that your baby will be born too early, weigh too much, or have breathing problems or low blood glucose right after birth.

About This Chapter: This chapter includes text excerpted from "Pregnancy If You Have Diabetes," National Institute of Diabetes and Digestive and Kidney Diseases (NIDDK), January 2017.

High blood glucose also can increase the chance that you will have a miscarriage or a stillborn baby. Stillborn means the baby dies in the womb during the second half of pregnancy.

An Extra Large Baby

Diabetes that is not well controlled causes the baby's blood sugar to be high. The baby is "overfed" and grows extra large. Besides causing discomfort to the woman during the last few months of pregnancy, an extra large baby can lead to problems during delivery for both the mother and the baby. The mother might need a C-Section to deliver the baby. The baby can be born with nerve damage due to pressure on the shoulder during delivery.

(Source: "Type 1 Or Type 2 Diabetes And Pregnancy," Centers for Disease Control and Prevention (CDC).)

How Can My Diabetes Affect Me During Pregnancy?

Hormonal and other changes in your body during pregnancy affect your blood glucose levels, so you might need to change how you manage your diabetes. Even if you've had diabetes for years, you may need to change your meal plan, physical activity routine, and medicines. If you have been taking an oral diabetes medicine, you may need to switch to insulin. As you get closer to your due date, your management plan might change again.

What Health Problems Could I Develop During Pregnancy Because Of My Diabetes?

Pregnancy can worsen certain long-term diabetes problems, such as eye problems and kidney disease, especially if your blood glucose levels are too high.

You also have a greater chance of developing preeclampsia, sometimes called toxemia, which is when you develop high blood pressure and too much protein in your urine during the second half of pregnancy. Preeclampsia can cause serious or life-threatening problems for you and your baby. The only cure for preeclampsia is to give birth. If you have preeclampsia and have reached 37 weeks of pregnancy, your doctor may want to deliver your baby early. Before 37 weeks, you and your doctor may consider other options to help your baby develop as much as possible before he or she is born.

How Can I Prepare For Pregnancy If I Have Diabetes?

If you have diabetes, keeping your blood glucose as close to normal as possible before and during your pregnancy is important to stay healthy and have a healthy baby. Getting checkups before and during pregnancy, following your diabetes meal plan, being physically active as your healthcare team advises, and taking diabetes medicines if you need to will help you manage your diabetes. Stopping smoking and taking vitamins as your doctor advises also can help you and your baby stay healthy.

Adjust Your Medicines

Some medicines are not safe during pregnancy and you should stop taking them before you get pregnant. Tell your doctor about all the medicines you take, such as those for high cholesterol and high blood pressure. Your doctor can tell you which medicines to stop taking, and may prescribe a different medicine that is safe to use during pregnancy.

Doctors most often prescribe insulin for both type 1 and type 2 diabetes during pregnancy. If you're already taking insulin, you might need to change the kind, the amount, or how and when you take it. You may need less insulin during your first trimester but probably will need more as you go through pregnancy. Your insulin needs may double or even triple as you get closer to your due date. Your healthcare team will work with you to create an insulin routine to meet your changing needs.

Take Vitamin And Mineral Supplements

Folic acid is an important vitamin for you to take before and during pregnancy to protect your baby's health. You'll need to start taking folic acid at least 1 month before you get pregnant. You should take a multivitamin or supplement that contains at least 400 micrograms (mcg) of folic acid. Once you become pregnant, you should take 600 mcg daily.4 Ask your doctor if you should take other vitamins or minerals, such as iron or calcium supplements, or a multivitamin.

What Do I Need To Know About Blood Glucose Testing Before And During Pregnancy?

How often you check your blood glucose levels may change during pregnancy. You may need to check them more often than you do now. If you didn't need to check your blood glucose before pregnancy, you will probably need to start. Ask your healthcare team how often and at what times you should check your blood glucose levels. Your blood glucose targets will change during pregnancy. Your healthcare team also may want you to check your ketone levels if your blood glucose is too high.

Target Blood Glucose Levels Before Pregnancy

When you're planning to become pregnant, your daily blood glucose targets may be different than your previous targets. Ask your healthcare team which targets are right for you.

You can keep track of your blood glucose levels using My Daily Blood Glucose Record. You can also use an electronic blood glucose tracking system on your computer or mobile device. Record the results every time you check your blood glucose. Your blood glucose records can help you and your healthcare team decide whether your diabetes care plan is working. You also can make notes about your insulin and ketones. Take your tracker with you when you visit your healthcare team.

Target Blood Glucose Levels During Pregnancy

Recommended daily target blood glucose numbers for most pregnant women with diabetes are

- Before meals, at bedtime, and overnight: 90 or less

- 1 hour after eating: 130 to 140 or less

- 2 hours after eating: 120 or less

Ask your doctor what targets are right for you. If you have type 1 diabetes, your targets may be higher so you don't develop low blood glucose, also called hypoglycemia.

A1C Numbers

Another way to see whether you're meeting your targets is to have an A1C blood test. Results of the A1C test reflect your average blood glucose levels during the past 3 months. Most women with diabetes should aim for an A1C as close to normal as possible—ideally below 6.5 percent—before getting pregnant.[3] After the first 3 months of pregnancy, your target may be as low as 6 percent.[3] These targets may be different than A1C goals you've had in the past. Your doctor can help you set A1C targets that are best for you.

Ketone Levels

When your blood glucose is too high or if you're not eating enough, your body might make ketones. Ketones in your urine or blood mean your body is using fat for energy instead of glucose. Burning large amounts of fat instead of glucose can be harmful to your health and your baby's health.

You can prevent serious health problems by checking for ketones. Your doctor might recommend you test your urine or blood daily for ketones or when your blood glucose is above a certain level, such as 200. If you use an insulin pump, your doctor might advise you to test for ketones when your blood glucose level is higher than expected. Your healthcare team can teach you how and when to test your urine or blood for ketones.

Talk with your doctor about what to do if you have ketones. Your doctor might suggest making changes in the amount of insulin you take or when you take it. Your doctor also may recommend a change in meals or snacks if you need to consume more carbohydrates.

Tips For Women With Diabetes

1. See your doctor early and often
2. Eat healthy foods
3. Exercise regularly
4. Take pills and insulin as directed
5. Control and treat low blood sugar quickly
6. Monitor blood sugar often

(Source: "Type 1 Or Type 2 Diabetes And Pregnancy," Centers for Disease Control and Prevention (CDC).)

Chapter 40

Gestational Diabetes And Pregnancy

Gestational diabetes is a type of diabetes that is first seen in a pregnant woman who did not have diabetes before she was pregnant. Some women have more than one pregnancy affected by gestational diabetes. Gestational diabetes usually shows up in the middle of pregnancy. Doctors most often test for it between 24 and 28 weeks of pregnancy.

Often gestational diabetes can be controlled through eating healthy foods and regular exercise. Sometimes a woman with gestational diabetes must also take insulin.

Problems Of Gestational Diabetes In Pregnancy

Blood sugar that is not well controlled in a woman with gestational diabetes can lead to problems for the pregnant woman and the baby:

An Extra Large Baby

Diabetes that is not well controlled causes the baby's blood sugar to be high. The baby is "overfed" and grows extra large. Besides causing discomfort to the woman during the last few months of pregnancy, an extra large baby can lead to problems during delivery for both the mother and the baby. The mother might need a C-section to deliver the baby. The baby can be born with nerve damage due to pressure on the shoulder during delivery.

C-Section (Cesarean Section)

A C-section is an operation to deliver the baby through the mother's belly. A woman who has diabetes that is not well controlled has a higher chance of needing a C-section to deliver

About This Chapter: This chapter includes text excerpted from "Gestational Diabetes And Pregnancy," Centers for Disease Control and Prevention (CDC), September 16, 2015.

the baby. When the baby is delivered by a C-section, it takes longer for the woman to recover from childbirth.

High Blood Pressure (Preeclampsia)

When a pregnant woman has high blood pressure, protein in her urine, and often swelling in fingers and toes that doesn't go away, she might have preeclampsia. It is a serious problem that needs to be watched closely and managed by her doctor. High blood pressure can cause harm to both the woman and her unborn baby. It might lead to the baby being born early and also could cause seizures or a stroke (a blood clot or a bleed in the brain that can lead to brain damage) in the woman during labor and delivery. Women with diabetes have high blood pressure more often than women without diabetes.

Low Blood Sugar (Hypoglycemia)

People with diabetes who take insulin or other diabetes medications can develop blood sugar that is too low. Low blood sugar can be very serious, and even fatal, if not treated quickly. Seriously low blood sugar can be avoided if women watch their blood sugar closely and treat low blood sugar early.

If a woman's diabetes was not well controlled during pregnancy, her baby can very quickly develop low blood sugar after birth. The baby's blood sugar must be watched for several hours after delivery.

Gestational Diabetes And Problems To The Baby

- Injury during birth if the baby is very large
- Increased risk for developing type 2 diabetes later in life
- Stillbirth

(Source: "Check Your Knowledge: Diabetes And Pregnancy," Centers for Disease Control and Prevention (CDC).)

Tips For Women With Gestational Diabetes

1. Eat Healthy Foods

Eat healthy foods from a meal plan made for a person with diabetes. A dietitian can help you create a healthy meal plan. A dietitian can also help you learn how to control your blood sugar while you are pregnant.

Gestational Diabetes That Is Not Controlled Can Cause You To

- Have problems during delivery.
- Have a very large baby and need to have a Cesarean section (C-section) (an operation to get your baby out through your abdomen).
- Take longer to recover from childbirth if your baby is delivered by C-section.

(Source: "Diabetes And Pregnancy," Centers for Disease Control and Prevention (CDC).)

2. Exercise Regularly

Exercise is another way to keep blood sugar under control. It helps to balance food intake. After checking with your doctor, you can exercise regularly during and after pregnancy. Get at least 30 minutes of moderate-intensity physical activity at least five days a week. This could be brisk walking, swimming, or actively playing with children.

3. Monitor Blood Sugar Often

Because pregnancy causes the body's need for energy to change, blood sugar levels can change very quickly. Check your blood sugar often, as directed by your doctor.

4. Take Insulin, If Needed

Sometimes a woman with gestational diabetes must take insulin. If insulin is ordered by your doctor, take it as directed in order to help keep blood sugar under control.

5. Get Tested For Diabetes After Pregnancy

Get tested for diabetes 6 to 12 weeks after your baby is born, and then every 1 to 3 years.

For most women with gestational diabetes, the diabetes goes away soon after delivery. When it does not go away, the diabetes is called type 2 diabetes. Even if the diabetes does go away after the baby is born, half of all women who had gestational diabetes develop type 2 diabetes later. It's important for a woman who has had gestational diabetes to continue to exercise and eat a healthy diet after pregnancy to prevent or delay getting type 2 diabetes. She should also remind her doctor to check her blood sugar every 1 to 3 years.

Chapter 41
Preparing For Multiple Births

Over the past three decades, there's been a phenomenal rise in the number of multiple births in the United States. What's responsible for this dramatic rise in multiple births? And how should you prepare for your own multiple birth experience?

The Miracle Of Multiples

Several factors contribute to the development of a multiple pregnancy:

- **Heredity:** A history of multiple births on a woman's side of the family increases her chances of having a multiple pregnancy.

- **Race:** Women of African descent are the most likely to have multiple pregnancies.

- **Number of prior pregnancies:** Having more than one previous pregnancy, especially a multiple pregnancy, increases the chance of having a multiple pregnancy.

- **Delayed childbearing:** Older women who get pregnant are more likely to have multiples.

- **Infertility treatment:** Fertility drugs, which stimulate the ovaries to release multiple eggs, or assisted reproductive technology (ART), which may transfer multiple embryos into the womb (such as in vitro fertilization, or IVF), greatly increase a woman's chance of having a multiple pregnancy.

It's the last two factors that have been on the rise in the last couple of decades and are probably responsible for the increase in multiple births.

The Types Of Multiples

There are two types of twins: **monozygotic** (identical) and **dizygotic** (fraternal).

Identical twins result from a single fertilized egg dividing into separate halves and continuing to develop into two separate but identical babies. These twins are genetically identical, with the same chromosomes and similar physical characteristics. They're the same sex and have the same blood type, hair, and eye color.

Fraternal twins come from two eggs that are fertilized by two separate sperm and are no more alike than other siblings born to the same parents. They may or may not be the same sex. This type of twins is much more common, and only this type is affected by heredity, maternal age, race, and number of prior pregnancies.

"Supertwins" is a common term for triplets and other higher-order multiple births, such as quadruplets or quintuplets. These babies can be identical, fraternal, or a combination of both.

The Risks of Multiple Births

The most common risk involved with multiple births is pre-term (or early) labor resulting in premature births. A typical, single pregnancy lasts about 40 weeks, but a twin pregnancy often lasts between 35 to 37 weeks. More than half of all twins are born prematurely (before 37 weeks), and the risk of having a premature delivery increases with higher-order multiples.

Premature babies (preemies) can have numerous health challenges. Because the care of premature babies is so different from that of full-term infants, preemies are usually placed in a neonatal intensive care unit (NICU) after delivery. The risk of developing health problems increases with the degree of prematurity—babies born closer to their due date have a lower risk.

In addition to the possibility of premature births, other medical conditions that are more likely to occur during a multiple pregnancy include preeclampsia, gestational diabetes, placental problems, and fetal growth problems. Being part of a multiple birth can also be associated with long-term health problems in the infants. Developmental delays and cerebral palsy occur more commonly in twins than in single births, and there's a higher risk of enduring health problems with higher-order multiple births.

Because of these concerns, many doctors who specialize in fertility treatments require prospective parents to undergo intensive counseling on the possibilities and risks associated with multiple births.

Staying Healthy During A Multiple Pregnancy

Eating properly, getting enough rest, and making regular trips to the doctor are critical measures for any expectant mother to stay healthy. And a woman with a multiple pregnancy might be scheduled for more frequent appointments with her obstetrician/gynecologist (OB-GYN) than a women who is pregnant with a single fetus.

The need for frequent, intensive prenatal care is of the utmost importance in a multiple pregnancy. You'll want to be particularly careful about finding healthcare professionals who have experience with multiple births. Because multiple pregnancies are automatically termed high-risk, the need for specialized healthcare is vital to ensuring that you and your babies receive the best care available.

Because you may not know anyone who has experienced a multiple birth, asking for a referral from a friend may not be productive. Instead, ask your doctor or OB-GYN to recommend a facility that specializes in multiple births. You should be part of a pre-term birth prevention program at your hospital and have immediate access to a specialized NICU should you go into early labor or if one of your babies is born with a health problem.

Your Nutrition

If you're pregnant with multiples, you should follow general pregnancy nutrition guidelines, including increasing your calcium and folic acid intake. Pregnant women need additional calcium, so extra milk or fortified orange juice, broccoli, sardines, or other calcium-rich foods should be added to your diet.

As with all expectant mothers, folic acid is extremely important. Taking folic acid at least 1 month prior to and throughout the pregnancy will decrease the risk of neural tube defects (such as spina bifida).

Another dietary requirement that needs to be increased if you're expecting more than one baby is protein. Getting enough protein can help your babies grow properly.

During pregnancy, an increased supply of iron is also needed for hemoglobin, the substance in red blood cells that binds oxygen for delivery to the tissues. Not getting enough iron can lead to a condition known as iron-deficiency anemia. Anemia occurs when the number of healthy red blood cells decreases in the body), and is relatively common in multiple pregnancies.

Anemia can cause shortness of breath and extreme fatigue during a pregnancy, as well as a reduced oxygen supply to the developing babies. Your doctor will probably prescribe an iron supplement, as your requirement for this mineral usually can't be met by diet alone. Iron is absorbed more easily when combined with foods that have high amounts of vitamin C, like orange juice.

Additional fetuses also mean an increased need for all other nutrients (such as zinc, copper, vitamin C, and vitamin D). So it's important to take your prenatal vitamin supplement every day. But just because you're carrying more than one baby doesn't mean you should take more than one prenatal vitamin—one is enough and too much can even be harmful.

Your Weight

Mothers carrying multiples are expected to gain more weight during pregnancy than mothers carrying a single fetus. But exactly how much weight you should gain depends on your pre-pregnancy weight and the number of fetuses, so make sure to talk to your doctor.

In general, though, you should consume about 300 additional calories a day for each fetus. It might be tough to eat a lot when your abdomen is full of babies, so try to eat smaller, more frequent meals.

Your Comfort

Of course, expecting multiples means that you're probably experiencing the typical discomforts of pregnancy more intensely. Nurturing yourself can help ease the stress of pregnancy.

Expectant partners can help, too. Something as simple as having someone brush your hair can make the discomforts of pregnancy fade momentarily. It helps, too, if your partner remembers that your body is going through tremendous hormonal changes. Communication and understanding can be the keys to truly enjoying this special time in your lives.

Preparing For Childbirth

Getting ready for a multiple birth may seem overwhelming, and concerns about pre-term labor can be additional burdens for you to bear. The best reassurance is knowing that you have a network of support around you: capable doctors, a caring hospital staff, and a partner, family members, and/or friends.

To help you be more comfortable with the birth process as it unfolds, you should also discuss the options of vaginal delivery versus Cesarean section (C-section) with your doctor well before your due date. Several factors affect the safety of each approach. Even if you and your doctor agree to attempt a vaginal delivery, circumstances may arise during labor or delivery that make a C-section necessary.

You may choose to have additional birthing attendants in the room during labor and birth. For example, midwives are becoming more common. For multiples, it is usually recommended that a midwife work with a doctor, rather than alone. A certified nurse-midwife (CNM) has specialized training in midwifery and is registered or licensed in all 50 states.

Hiring a doula is another option. The term comes from ancient Greece, where the doula was the primary attendant to the female head of the household. Today, doulas offer support services to women during the birth, as well as after delivery, by assisting with infant care and household chores.

Special Delivery

As labor begins, you'll likely be connected to a fetal monitor so your doctor can check each baby's progress. The interval between the birth of each baby delivered vaginally is usually less than 20 to 30 minutes. And here's one piece of good news: Because multiple-birth babies tend to be smaller than single ones, it's easier to push them out. Luckily, they only come out one at a time!

In the case of multiples, though, a vaginal delivery may not always be possible. The crowded uterus can cause compression of the placenta or umbilical cord of any of the soon-to-be-born babies during labor. Prolonged compression may put one or more babies at serious risk as labor progresses during attempts at vaginal delivery. So prompt delivery by C-section may be necessary in these cases.

Positioning of the babies can also affect the safety of a vaginal delivery. It's common for the first baby to be born head first, whereas the subsequent infants may be breech (buttocks or feet first), transverse (sideways), or head first when entering the birth canal. Usually, if the first fetus is not head first, the babies will be delivered by C-section. And most triplets and other higher-order multiples are born by C-section.

If your doctor needs to perform a C-section, a catheter will be placed in your bladder, you'll be given anesthesia, and an incision will be made in your abdomen and uterus. The doctor will then deliver your babies through the incision. The babies will be delivered within just a few minutes of each other with this approach.

If you go into labor prematurely, you and your unborn babies will be closely monitored for signs of distress. You may have to make decisions on the delivery method and procedures at this time, so consider your options before arriving at the hospital.

Many babies born prematurely will need to go immediately to the NICU for the special care they need. Visitations by family members are usually encouraged, often right from the first day.

Taking Your Babies Home

The first days, weeks, and months are often the most difficult for parents of multiples, as everyone learns to get used to the frequent feedings, lack of sleep, and little personal time involved in parenting multiples.

It can help to join a support group for parents of multiples. Hearing what has worked well for others can help you find solutions to problems you come across.

Enlist whatever help you can get—from neighbors, family members, and friends—for household chores and daily tasks. Having extra hands around can not only make feedings easier and help you rest and recover from delivery, it can also give you the precious time you need to get to know your babies.

Chapter 42

Miscarriage And Stillbirth

Pregnancy Loss / Miscarriage

What Is Pregnancy Loss / Miscarriage?

A miscarriage, also called pregnancy loss or spontaneous abortion, is the unexpected loss of a fetus before the 20th week of pregnancy, or gestation. (Gestation is the period of pregnancy from conception to birth.) The loss of a pregnancy after the 20th week of gestation is called a stillbirth and can occur before or during delivery.

What Are The Symptoms Of Pregnancy Loss / Miscarriage?

Symptoms of miscarriage may include vaginal spotting or bleeding; abdominal pain or abdominal cramps; low back pain; or fluid, tissue, or clot-like material passing from the vagina. Although vaginal bleeding is a common symptom when a woman has a miscarriage, many pregnant women have spotting early during their pregnancy because of other factors but do not miscarry. Regardless, pregnant women who have any of the symptoms of miscarriage should contact their healthcare providers immediately.

How Many People Are Affected By Or At Risk For Pregnancy Loss / Miscarriage?

The estimated rate of miscarriage is 15 percent to 20 percent in women who know they are pregnant, but as many as half of all fertilized eggs may spontaneously abort, often before the

About This Chapter: Text under the heading "Pregnancy Loss / Miscarriage" is excerpted from "Pregnancy Loss: Condition Information," *Eunice Kennedy Shriver* National Institute of Child Health and Human Development (NICHD), December 4, 2012. Reviewed March 2017; Text under the heading "Stillbirth" is excerpted from "Facts About Stillbirth," Centers for Disease Control and Prevention (CDC), October 12, 2016.

women realize they are pregnant. Women who have had previous miscarriages are at a higher risk for miscarriage. The risk of miscarriage also increases with maternal age beginning at age 30 and becoming greater after age 35.

What Causes Pregnancy Loss / Miscarriage?

Miscarriage occurs due to many different causes, some of them known and others unknown. Frequently, miscarriages occur when a pregnancy is not developing normally. More than half of all miscarriages are caused by a chromosomal abnormality in the fetus (typically due to the wrong number of chromosomes, the structures in a cell that contain the genetic information), which is more common with increasing age of the parents, particularly among women who are older than age 35.

Other possible causes of pregnancy loss or miscarriage are maternal health issues or exposure to chemicals. Maternal health issues include chronic disease, such as diabetes, thyroid disease, or polycystic ovary syndrome (PCOS), or problems associated with the immune system, such as an autoimmune disorder. Other maternal health issues that can increase the risk of miscarriage include infection, hormone problems, obesity, or problems of the placenta, cervix, or uterus. Exposure to environmental toxins, drug use or alcohol use, smoking, or the consumption of 200 milligrams or more of caffeine per day (equal to about one 12-ounce cup of coffee) also can increase the risk of miscarriage.

How Do Healthcare Providers Diagnose Pregnancy Loss / Miscarriage?

If a pregnant woman experiences any of the symptoms of miscarriage, such as crampy abdominal or back pain, light spotting, or bleeding, she should contact her healthcare provider immediately. For diagnosis, the woman may need to undergo a blood test to check for the level of hCG, the pregnancy hormone, or an internal pelvic examination to determine if her cervix is dilated or thinned, which can be a sign of a miscarriage; or depending on the length of time since her last menstrual period, and the level of pregnancy hormone in the blood, she may need to have an ultrasound test so that her healthcare provider can observe the pregnancy and the maternal reproductive organs, such as the uterus and placenta. If a woman has had more than one miscarriage, she may choose to have blood tests performed to check for chromosome abnormalities or hormone problems, or to detect immune system disorders that may interfere with a healthy pregnancy.

What Are The Treatments For Pregnancy Loss / Miscarriage?

In most cases, no treatment is necessary for women who miscarry early in their pregnancy, because the bleeding associated with miscarriage usually empties the uterus of pregnancy-associated tissue. In some cases, however, a woman may need to undergo a surgical procedure called a dilation and curettage (D&C) to remove any pregnancy-associated tissue remaining in the uterus. A D&C is performed if the woman is bleeding heavily or if an ultrasound test detects any remaining tissue in the uterus.

An alternative to a D&C is the use of a medication called misoprostol that helps the tissue pass out of the uterus. The use of misoprostol has proven to be effective in 84 percent of the cases studied. Other treatments after a woman miscarries may include control of mild to moderate bleeding, prevention of infection, pain relief, and emotional support. If heavy bleeding occurs, the woman should contact her healthcare provider immediately.

Is There A Cure For Pregnancy Loss / Miscarriage?

In many cases, a woman can do little to prevent a miscarriage. However, having preconception and prenatal care (before becoming pregnant and during pregnancy) is the best prevention available for all complications associated with pregnancy. Miscarriages caused by systemic disease often can be prevented by detection and treatment of the disease before pregnancy occurs. A woman also can decrease her risk of miscarriage by avoiding environmental hazards, such as infectious diseases, X-rays, drugs and alcohol, and high levels of caffeine.

Stillbirth

What Is Stillbirth?

A stillbirth is the death of a baby before or during delivery. Both miscarriage and stillbirth are terms describing pregnancy loss, but they differ according to when the loss occurs. There is no universally accepted definition of when a fetal death is called a stillbirth, and the meaning of this term varies internationally. This lack of a consistent definition of stillbirth often makes it difficult to compare data on how frequently it occurs.

In the United States, a miscarriage usually refers to a fetal loss less than 20 weeks after a woman becomes pregnant, and a stillbirth refers to a loss 20 or more weeks after a woman becomes pregnant.

Stillbirth is further classified as either early, late, or term.

- An early stillbirth is a fetal death occurring between 20 and 27 completed weeks of pregnancy.

- A late stillbirth occurs between 28 and 36 completed pregnancy weeks.

- A term stillbirth occurs between 37 or more completed pregnancy weeks.

Occurrence

Stillbirth effects about 1 percent of all pregnancies, and each year about 24,000 babies are stillborn in the United States. That is about the same number of babies that die during the first year of life and it is more than 10 times as many deaths as the number that occur from Sudden Infant Death Syndrome (SIDS).

Because of advances in medical technology over the last 30 years, prenatal care (medical care during pregnancy) has improved, which has dramatically reduced the number of late and term stillbirth. However, the rate of early stillbirth has remained about the same over time.

Causes

The causes of many stillbirths are unknown. Therefore, families are often left grieving without answers to their questions. Stillbirth is not a cause of death, but rather a term that means a baby's death during the pregnancy. Some women blame themselves, but rarely are these deaths caused by something a woman did or did not do. Known causes of stillbirth generally fall into one of three broad categories:

- Problems with the baby (birth defects or genetic problems)

- Problems with the placenta or umbilical cord (this is where the mother and baby exchange oxygen and nutrients)

- Certain conditions in the mother (for example, uncontrolled diabetes, high blood pressure, or obesity)

Stillbirth with an unknown cause is called "unexplained stillbirth." Having an unexplained stillbirth is more likely to occur the further along a woman is in her pregnancy.

Although stillbirth occurs in families of all races, ethnicities, and income levels, and to women of all ages, some women are at higher risk for having a stillbirth. Some of the factors that increase the risk for a stillbirth include the mother:

- being of black race

- being a teenager

- being 35 years of age or older

- being unmarried

- being obese

- smoking cigarettes during pregnancy

- having certain medical conditions, such as high blood pressure or diabetes

- having multiple pregnancies

- having had a previous pregnancy loss

These factors are also associated with other poor pregnancy outcomes, such as preterm birth.

What Can Be Done?

Although many causes of stillbirth remain unknown, more causes might be found if thorough investigations were performed, including an autopsy (a physical exam of a body after death), placental exam, genetic testing, and a detailed medical history. This information can be important in finding out whether there is a chance that a stillbirth could occur again and to provide appropriate medical care and counseling for future pregnancies. Even when a cause is not found, many families report that having an evaluation and looking for a cause was helpful in coping with their loss. After a stillbirth occurs, physicians can help by looking for a specific cause and arranging for grief counseling for the mother and family.

Part Five
Childbirth

Chapter 43
Your Developing Baby

First Trimester (Week 1–Week 12)

At Four Weeks

- Your baby's brain and spinal cord have begun to form.

- The heart begins to form.

- Arm and leg buds appear.

- Your baby is now an embryo and one-twenty-fifth inch long.

At Eight Weeks

- All major organs and external body structures have begun to form.

- Your baby's heart beats with a regular rhythm.

- The arms and legs grow longer, and fingers and toes have begun to form.

- The sex organs begin to form.

- The eyes have moved forward on the face and eyelids have formed.

- The umbilical cord is clearly visible.

- At the end of eight weeks, your baby is a fetus and looks more like a human. Your baby is nearly 1 inch long and weighs less than one-eighth ounce.

About This Chapter: This chapter includes text excerpted from "Stages Of Pregnancy," Office on Women's Health (OWH), U.S. Department of Health and Human Services (HHS), September 27, 2010. Reviewed March 2017.

At 12 Weeks

- The nerves and muscles begin to work together. Your baby can make a fist.

- The external sex organs show if your baby is a boy or girl. A woman who has an ultrasound in the second trimester or later might be able to find out the baby's sex.

- Eyelids close to protect the developing eyes. They will not open again until the 28th week.

- Head growth has slowed, and your baby is much longer. Now, at about 3 inches long, your baby weighs almost an ounce.

Second Trimester (Week 13–Week 28)

At 16 Weeks

- Muscle tissue and bone continue to form, creating a more complete skeleton.

- Skin begins to form. You can nearly see through it.

- Meconium develops in your baby's intestinal tract. This will be your baby's first bowel movement.

- Your baby makes sucking motions with the mouth (sucking reflex).

- Your baby reaches a length of about 4 to 5 inches and weighs almost 3 ounces.

At 20 Weeks

Your baby is more active. You might feel slight fluttering.

- Your baby is covered by fine, downy hair called lanugo and a waxy coating called vernix. This protects the forming skin underneath.

- Eyebrows, eyelashes, fingernails, and toenails have formed. Your baby can even scratch itself.

- Your baby can hear and swallow.

- Now halfway through your pregnancy, your baby is about 6 inches long and weighs about 9 ounces.

At 24 Weeks

- Bone marrow begins to make blood cells.

- Taste buds form on your baby's tongue.

- Footprints and fingerprints have formed.
- Real hair begins to grow on your baby's head.
- The lungs are formed, but do not work.
- The hand and startle reflex develop.
- Your baby sleeps and wakes regularly.
- If your baby is a boy, his testicles begin to move from the abdomen into the scrotum. If your baby is a girl, her uterus and ovaries are in place, and a lifetime supply of eggs have formed in the ovaries.
- Your baby stores fat and has gained quite a bit of weight. Now at about 12 inches long, your baby weighs about 1½ pounds.

Third Trimester (Week 29–Week 40)

At 32 Weeks

- Your baby's bones are fully formed, but still soft.
- Your baby's kicks and jabs are forceful.
- The eyes can open and close and sense changes in light.
- Lungs are not fully formed, but practice "breathing" movements occur.
- Your baby's body begins to store vital minerals, such as iron and calcium.
- Lanugo begins to fall off.
- Your baby is gaining weight quickly, about one-half pound a week. Now, your baby is about 15 to 17 inches long and weighs about 4 to 4½ pounds.

At 36 Weeks

- The protective waxy coating called vernix gets thicker.
- Body fat increases. Your baby is getting bigger and bigger and has less space to move around. Movements are less forceful, but you will feel stretches and wiggles.
- Your baby is about 16 to 19 inches long and weighs about 6 to 6½ pounds.

Weeks 37–40

- By the end of 37 weeks, your baby is considered full term. Your baby's organs are ready to function on their own.

- As you near your due date, your baby may turn into a head-down position for birth. Most babies "present" head down.

- At birth, your baby may weigh somewhere between 6 pounds 2 ounces and 9 pounds 2 ounces and be 19 to 21 inches long. Most full-term babies fall within these ranges. But healthy babies come in many different sizes.

- Infants born before 37 weeks are considered preterm. These children are at increased risk for problems such as developmental delays, vision and hearing problems, and cerebral palsy.
- Infants born in the 37th and 38th weeks of pregnancy—previously considered full term—are now considered "early term." These infants face more health risks than infants who are born at 39 weeks or later.
- Infants born at 39 or 40 weeks of pregnancy are considered full term. Full-term infants have better health outcomes than do infants born earlier or, in some cases, later than this period. Therefore, if the mother and baby are healthy, it is best to deliver at or after 39 weeks to give the infant's lungs, brain, and liver time to fully develop.
- Infants born at 41 weeks through 41 weeks and 6 days are considered late term.
- Infants who are born at 42 weeks and beyond are considered postterm.

(Source:"Pregnancy: Condition Information," Eunice Kennedy Shriver *National Institute of Child Health and Human Development (NICHD).)*

Chapter 44
Items Your Baby Will Need

Many parents-to-be enjoy putting together their baby's layette. This is the clothing and supplies your baby will need in the months ahead. There are countless baby items, and every gadget comes in different shapes, sizes, and brands. So, it can be hard to know what items you will really need or use.

The list that follows will give you some ideas about what you might need and want. Ask mothers you know about what items they couldn't live without and brands they liked. Also, keep in mind that the cost of brand-new baby gear can add up. Many new parents keep costs down by borrowing clothes and gear or shopping at consignment stores.

Safety is also an important factor when shopping for supplies. Some products may pose a risk to your baby if safety guidelines are not followed. And used products are more likely than new items to be dangerous.

What Your Baby Will Need At The Hospital

- Undershirt
- An outfit such as a stretch suit, nightgown, or sweater set
- A pair of socks or booties
- Receiving blanket, cap, and heavier blanket or bunting, if the weather is cold
- Diapers and wipes (some hospitals provide an initial supply of these)
- Infant car seat

About This Chapter: This chapter includes text excerpted from "Baby's Layette," Office on Women's Health (OWH), U.S. Department of Health and Human Services (HHS), September 27, 2010. Reviewed March 2017.

Things You'll Need To Transport Your Baby

- Rear-facing infant car seat—A proper car seat is the best way to protect your baby on the road and the only legal way to transport your baby in a car. Buying a new seat is best, so that you can be sure the seat is safe and in good condition. Be careful when using an infant car seat outside the car. Do not place a car seat holding a baby on table tops or other elevated surfaces. Improper use of car seats outside the car puts babies at risk of injury and death. Common reasons for car seat-related injuries include falling out of car seats, car seats falling from elevated surfaces, and car seats overturning on soft surfaces.

- Stroller

- Soft carrier, sling, or backpack

- Diaper bag—since this is something you will be carrying around for about three years, choose one that is comfortable and durable for you.

Items For Your Baby's Room

- Crib and crib linens—Most brand new cribs and mattresses purchased in the United States are safe. If you are planning to use a used crib, make sure it conforms to the current government safety standards. Do not use infant sleep positioners, which are dangerous and not needed.

- Play pen or portable crib

- Changing table

- Dresser

- Glider or rocking chair

- Clothes hamper

- Baby monitor

- Night light/soft lighting

Most hospitals will not discharge the baby unless the car seat is checked for safety and correct installation.

Infant Care Items

- Diapers or cloth diapers—you can get a couple of different brands of diapers so you can test them out and choose your favorite.

- Receiving blankets

- Clothing

- Breast pump (if you plan to breastfeed)

- Bottles—be sure to get the correct size of nipples, such as preemie, or newborn.

- Rectal or digital ear thermometer

- Bathtub

- Washcloths and baby wipes

- Diaper rash ointment and/or petroleum jelly

- Hooded towels

- Diaper disposal system—good to have, but not necessary.

- Burp cloths and waterproof lap pads

- Bulb syringe—for suctioning baby's nasal passages if necessary. Your baby's doctor will tell you if, when, and how to do this.

- Baby nail clippers/scissors manicure set

Things You'll Need As Your Baby Gets Older

- Outlet covers, cabinet locks, and other items to "childproof" your home

- Toys

- Books

- High chair

- Gates

Chapter 45
Making Your Home Safe For Baby

Your baby is on the way, and there is a lot to think about. Besides making sure that you have baby furniture and clothing for your new son or daughter, you'll want to check that your home is safe. These tips can help you cover all the safety bases.

Before You Bring Your Baby Home

- **Check the safety of your baby's crib and other baby items.** Many new parents welcome hand-me-down baby items from family and friends. Although it's wise to save money, some products could be unsafe if recalled or if parts are missing or loose. Unsafe cribs and other items can put your baby's life in danger. Most brand new cribs and mattresses purchased in the United States are safe. Make sure the crib conforms to the current government safety standards. Also, check to see if hand-me-down items, such as bassinets or portable cribs, have been recalled.

- **Remove pillows, blankets, and stuffed animals from the crib to prevent your baby from suffocation.**

- **Check to see that smoke detectors and carbon monoxide detectors in your home are working.** Place at least one smoke detector on each level of your home and in halls outside of bedrooms. Have an escape plan in case of fire.

About This Chapter: Text in this chapter begins with excerpts from "Making Your Home Safe For Baby," Office on Women's Health (OWH), U.S. Department of Health and Human Services (HHS), September 27, 2010. Reviewed March 2017; Text under the heading "Baby Safety Checklist" is excerpted from "Baby Safety Checklist," U.S. Consumer Product Safety Commission (CPSC), November 21, 2008. Reviewed March 2017.

- **Put emergency numbers, including poison control, near each phone.** Have at least one phone in your home connected by land line. Cordless phones do not work when the power is out, and cellphone batteries can run out.

- **Make sure your home or apartment number is easy to see so fire or rescue can locate you quickly in an emergency.**

- **Make sure handrails are installed and secure in stairways.** Always hold the handrail when using stairs, especially when holding your baby.

Before Your Baby Starts Crawling

Your baby will be crawling before you know it. Most babies begin crawling around six to nine months. Crawling on your hands and knees will reveal many dangers to your baby. Thinking ahead to the toddler years will help you to take care of other hazards before your baby grows and finds them first. Here are some things to do before your baby is crawling:

- Cover all unused electrical sockets with outlet plugs.

- Keep cords out of baby's reach. Tack up cords to vertical blinds and move furniture, lamps, or electronics to hide cords.

- Secure furniture and electronics, such as bookcases and TVs, so they cannot be pulled down on top of your baby.

- Use protective padding to cover sharp edges and corners, such as from a coffee table or fireplace hearth.

- Install safety gates at the bottom and top of stairwells or to block entry to unsafe rooms.

- Use safety latches on cabinets and doors.

- Store all medicines, cleaning products, and other poisons out of baby's reach.

- Remove rubber tips from doorstops or replace with one-piece doorstops.

- Look for and remove all small objects. Objects that easily can pass through the center of a toilet paper roll might cause choking.

- Keep houseplants out of baby's reach. Some plants can poison or make your baby sick.

- Set your water heater temperature to no higher than 125 degrees Fahrenheit. Water that is hotter can cause bad burns.

- Closely supervise your baby around a family pet. Pets need time to adjust to a new baby.

Baby Safety Checklist

Bathroom

- Never, ever, leave your child alone or under the supervision of a sibling in bathtub or near any water. Children can drown in only a few inches of water in seconds. Remember: bath seats or rings or other bathing aids are not safety devices.

- Keep medicines and cleaning products with child resistant lids locked and out of reach of children.

Kitchen

- Do not leave baby alone in a high chair and always use all safety straps. This will prevent injuries and deaths from the baby climbing out or from falling through leg openings.

- Keep matches, lighters, knives, and cleaning products with child resistant lids, locked and out of reach of children.

- Do not place your baby in any child or infant seat, including car seat carriers, infant carriers, bouncers, vibrating seats, or unsecured booster type chairs, on a countertop, table or any elevated surface. The baby's movements can cause the seat to fall, resulting in head or other injuries.

Around The house

- Use safety gates to block stairways and other dangerous areas. Avoid older gates that can collapse and entrap babies.

- Keep small objects, especially spherical toys such as marbles and objects with rounded ends away from children. These objects present a very high risk of choking.

- Keep toys with magnets away from young children. If two or more magnets are swallowed they can attract through intestinal walls and can cause holes, blockage, and infection which can result in death.

- If swallowed, un-inflated balloons and balloon pieces can lead to death by clinging to the airways.

- To avoid falls, secure windows with window guards.

- Secure furniture to avoid tip-overs.

Chapter 46
Taking Classes To Prepare For Baby

First-time mothers-to-be often have lots of questions and even some worries: How will I know I'm in labor? Will it hurt? Will my baby know how to breastfeed? How do I care for a newborn? Classes to prepare you for childbirth, breastfeeding, infant care, and parenting are great ways to lessen anxiety and build confidence. In some cities, classes might be offered in different languages.

Birthing Classes

Birthing classes often are offered through local hospitals and birthing centers. Some classes follow a specific method, such as Lamaze or the Bradley method. Others review labor techniques from a variety of methods. You might want to read about the different methods beforehand to see if one appeals more to you than others. That way, you will know what to sign up for if more than one type of birthing class if offered. Try to sign up for a class several months before your due date. Classes sometimes fill up quickly. Also, make sure the instructor is qualified.

Most women attend the class with the person who will provide support during labor, such as a spouse, sister, or good friend. This person is sometimes called the labor coach. During class, the instructor will go over the signs of labor and review the stages of labor. She will talk about positioning for labor and birth, and ways to control pain. She also will give you strategies to work through labor pains and to help you stay relaxed and in control. You will practice many

About This Chapter: Text in this chapter begins with excerpts from "Birthing, Breastfeeding, And Parenting Classes," Office on Women's Health (OWH), U.S. Department of Health and Human Services (HHS), September 27, 2010. Reviewed March 2017; Text beginning with the heading "Preparing For Emergency Birth" is excerpted from "Information For Pregnant Women," Centers for Disease Control and Prevention (CDC), January 31, 2014.

of these strategies in class, so you are ready when the big day arrives. Many classes also provide a tour of the birthing facility.

Breastfeeding Classes

Like any new skill, breastfeeding takes knowledge and practice to be successful. Pregnant women who learn about how to breastfeed are more likely to be successful than those who do not. Breastfeeding classes offer pregnant women and their partners the chance to prepare and ask questions before the baby's arrival. Classes may be offered through hospitals, breastfeeding support programs, La Leche League, or local lactation consultants. Ask your doctor for help finding a breastfeeding class in your area.

Parenting Classes

Many first-time parents have never cared for a newborn. Hospitals, community education centers, and places of worship sometimes offer baby care classes. These classes cover the basics, such as diapering, feeding, and bathing your newborn. You also will learn these basic skills in the hospital before you are discharged.

In some communities parenting classes are available. Children don't come with how-to manuals. So some parents appreciate learning about the different stages of child development, as well as practical skills for dealing with common issues, such as discipline or parent-child power struggles. Counselors and social workers often teach this type of class. If you are interested in parenting programs, ask your child's doctor for help finding a class in your area.

Preparing For Emergency Birth

Many childbirth education classes cover emergency birth procedures, with special attention to local resources.

- Work with your healthcare provide to learn the signs of early labor or other indications that may require assistance.

- Take a class on infant and child life support, offered by the American Red Cross (ARC) or the American Heart Association (AHA).

- Have a kit of emergency supplies in your home; such as, clean towels, sheets, clean scissors, sterile gloves, sanitary pads, diapers, and instructions for infant-rescue breathing

- Learn more about preparing for an emergency birth from the American College of Nurse-Midwives (ACNM).

Preparing For An Emergency Or Disaster

Find out what your local community action plan is, and what they recommend you do in an emergency situation. Every disaster is different and may require you to respond differently. (i.e., Do I evacuate? How should I evacuate? What is the nearest evacuation route? What if they tell me to stay at home or "shelter-in-place?")

- Talk to your healthcare provider about—

  - What you should do in any emergency.

  - Where you will get prenatal care.

  - Where you will deliver your baby if your hospital is closed.

- Make a back-up plan for getting to the hospital or healthcare center.

- Make an emergency plan.

  - Plan the steps you should take during an emergency. Ask your local American Red Cross for information on what they suggest every family prepare to do. Then develop your own plan, writing down the steps on paper.

  - Talk about potential disasters and emergencies and how to respond to each using your family plan. Choose a meeting place, other than your home, for family to gather in case you can't go home.

  - Give this emergency plan to all your family members. Have a family talk and give them a copy. Leave a copy in a prominent place in case other adults (e.g., babysitters) are in your home during an emergency.

  - Choose someone outside your home who can be an "emergency check-in" person in case someone cannot reach you or your family. Keep this person's telephone number and address with your plan and first aid kit. Give this number to friends and family members, including any children.

- Keep emergency supplies in your home to meet your family needs for at least three days. This includes the following:

  - **Water.** Each person needs 1 gallon of water each day.

  - **Food.** Store canned foods such as soups, beans, vegetables, fruit and juices, peanut butter, etc. Keep a non-electric can opener ready. If you have pets, stock up on dry or canned pet food.

- **Personal-care.** Store soap, toothpaste, contact lens solution, feminine hygiene products, nursing pads, clothes, etc.

- **Baby care.** The Centers for Disease Control and Prevention (CDC) and the American Academy of Pediatrics (AAP) recommend breastfeeding for optimal infant nutrition. Breastfeeding remains the best infant feeding option in a natural disaster situation. Even when experiencing diarrhea, food-borne illness, or extreme stress, breastfeeding mothers continue to produce ample milk for their babies. Also store baby supplies such as diapers, wipes, baby food, bottles, etc.

- **First aid kit that is custom-made for your family and the risks that you might encounter.**

- **Other supplies.** Make sure you have large plastic bags that seal for water-proofing important papers, a battery-powered flashlight and radio with extra batteries or a wind-up radio, and a first-aid kit.

- **If you cannot afford some of these items, ask for assistance from local emergency preparedness programs.**

- Gather important documents and information

  - Make copies of important records you need to prove your identity and that of family members.

  - Know what financial papers or items you will need and how to keep them safe (e.g., cash, ATM/EBT card, traveler's checks, long distance telephone cards, credit cards, checks).

  - Keep important contact information, toll-free numbers, and Websites together so you can learn about the status of the disaster, know where to get assistance, identify maternal and infant health resources, hospitals, etc.

  - Put "ICE" (In Case of Emergency) before important numbers on portable and cell phones. This helps emergency workers find the right person to contact in case of emergencies.

- Take every emergency or weather warning (e.g., tornado horn or severe weather alert) seriously. Use these alerts to test your family's emergency evacuation plan, equipment, and supplies (e.g., expiration dates, etc.).

Chapter 47
Creating Your Birth Plan

The birth of your baby should be one of the most memorable, life-changing, and joyful experiences of your life. You will want to spend time thinking through the details of your hopes and desires for this special event.

Starting with a journal, write down as many thoughts and plans for the upcoming birth as you can. Your journal will help you establish priorities and provide a list of ideas to help you create a birth plan.

A birth plan is a simple, clear, one-page statement of your preferences for the birth of your child. Providing a copy of the plan for everyone directly involved in the birth will help them better understand what is happening and give them the opportunity to resolve issues before the big day. Because there are so many aspects of birth to consider, it is best not to wait until the last minute to put your plan together.

The plan will provide an effective avenue for discussing important details with those responsible for supporting and caring for you.

Try to remain reasonably flexible in your desires because things don't always go according to plan. Remember, the important thing is the safe birth of your little bundle of joy.

Compile Considerations

Find out ALL the routine policies and procedures for "mommy care" in your birth setting. If you do not agree with a policy or procedure, you should discuss it with your healthcare

About This Chapter: Text in this chapter is excerpted from "Creating Your Birth Plan," © 2017 American Pregnancy Association. Reprinted with permission.

provider. As you learn more about what to expect, you will likely identify details that you want to include in your plan.

You may want to consider dedicating an entire page for an uncomplicated birth/postpartum and a second page about how to handle complications should they occur. The following list of questions might seem overwhelming, but now is the time to consider them one by one.

If you find that a question does not pertain to you, just move on to those that are relevant.

- Who do you want to be present?

- Do you want a doula?

- Will there be children/siblings present?

- Are you wishing to delay the cord clamping for baby?

- Do you want immediate skin to skin contact?

- Do you wish to breastfeed immediately after birth?

- Do you want mobility, or do you wish to stay in bed?

- What activities or positions do you plan to use? (walking, standing, squatting, hands and knees)

- Do you prefer a certain position to give birth?

- What will you do for pain relief? (massage, hot and cold packs, positions, labor imagery, relaxation, breathing exercises, tub or Jacuzzi, medication)

- How do you feel about fetal monitoring?

- How do you plan to stay hydrated? (sips of drinks, ice chips, IV)

- Do you want to take pain medications, or not? Do you have a preference for certain pain medications?

- Would you be willing to have an episiotomy? Or, are there certain measures you want to use to avoid one?

- What are your preferences for your baby's care? (when to feed, where to sleep)

- Do you want a routine IV, a heparin/saline block, or neither?

- Do you want to wear your own clothing?

- Do you want to listen to music and have focal points?

- Do you want to use the tub or shower?

- For home and birth center births, what are your plans for hospital transport in case of emergency?

- If you need a Cesarean, do you have any special requests?

Consult Your Healthcare Provider

Most of the time, healthcare providers have a set routine. They have been trained, and they also want what is best for the birth. Your healthcare provider may or may not be receptive to some of your ideas. They might view your list as being too demanding or as increasing certain risks.

Keeping in mind that every birth is different and that the definition of a "normal" birth can vary, try to use terms and phrases like "birth preferences," "our wishes for childbirth," "as long as birth progresses normally," or "unless there is an emergency." Make an appointment with the labor and birth department of your hospital or birthing center to have the staff review your plan in order to make suggestions.

You can request to spend time in an empty birthing or labor room to become more familiar with where you will be and what you might want to add to your packing list (extra pillows, pictures, music, etc). This should leave you feeling more confident about your birth plan and your choice of a birth location.

Confidence And Control

During childbirth, many women feel like they are losing control. A birth plan can help you maintain your focus and help you stay calm even if unexpected events occur.

Try to plan for the unexpected by using phrases like, "If a Cesarean becomes necessary…." During birth, if you feel pressured to do something about which you are uncertain, you can ask if it is an emergency situation. You can also request more information on any aspect of the situation and time to think about it.

The Power Of Positive Thinking

Design your birth plan with a positive focus. Instead of making a list of what you don't want, focus on what you do want. Use phrases like, "we hope to," "we plan to," or "we antici-pate." Try to avoid phrases like, "we don't want" or "we want to avoid."

Here are some examples:

- "Regarding pain management, I have studied and fully understand the types of pain medications available. I will ask for them if I need them."

- "Regarding an episiotomy, I am hoping to protect the perineum. I am practicing ahead of time by squatting, doing Kegel exercises, and perineal massage. I would appreciate guidance in when to push and when to stop pushing so the perineum can stretch."

- "Immediately following the birth, I plan to keep the baby near me. I would appreciate that the evaluation of the baby be done with the baby on my abdomen and with both of us covered by a warm blanket unless there is an unusual situation."

Chapter 48
Birthing Centers And Hospital Maternity Services

You'll make plenty of decisions during pregnancy, and choosing where to give birth—whether in a hospital or in a birth center setting—is one of the most important.

Hospitals

Many women fear that a hospital setting will be cold and clinical, but that's not necessarily true. A hospital setting can accommodate a variety of birth experiences.

Traditional hospital births (in which the mother-to-be moves from a labor room to a delivery room and then, after the birth, to a semiprivate room) are still the most common option. Doctors "manage" the delivery with their patients. In many cases, women in labor are not allowed to eat or drink for medical reasons, and they may be required to deliver in a certain position.

Pain medications are available during labor and delivery (if the woman chooses); labor may be induced, if necessary; and the fetus is usually electronically monitored throughout the labor. A birth plan can help a woman communicate her preferences about these issues, and doctors will abide by these as much possible.

In response to a push for more "natural" birth events, many hospitals now offer more modern options for low-risk births, often known as family-centered care. These may include private rooms with baths (birthing suites) where women can labor, deliver, and recover in one place without having to be moved.

Although a doctor and medical staff are still present, the rooms are usually set up to create a nurturing environment, with warm, soothing colors and features that try to simulate a home-like atmosphere that can be very comforting for new moms. Rooming in—when the baby stays with the mother most of the time instead of in the infant nursery—also may be available.

In addition, many hospitals offer childbirth and prenatal education classes to prepare parents for the birth experience and parenting classes for after the birth.

The number of people allowed to attend the birth varies from hospital to hospital. In more traditional settings, as many as three support people are permitted to be with the mother during a vaginal birth. In a family-centered approach, more family members, friends, and sometimes even kids might be allowed. During a routine or nonemergency C-section, usually just one support person allowed.

Hospital Births

If you decide to give birth in a hospital, you will see a variety of health professionals:

Obstetrician/gynecologists (OB/GYNs) are doctors with at least 4 additional years of training after medical school in women's health and reproduction, including both surgical and medical care. They can handle complicated pregnancies and also perform C-sections.

Look for obstetricians who are board-certified, meaning they have passed an examination by the American Board of Obstetrics and Gynecology (ACOG). Board-certified obstetricians who go on to receive further training in high-risk pregnancies are called **maternal-fetal specialists** or perinatologists.

If you deliver in a hospital, you also might be able to use a **certified nurse-midwife** (CNM). CNMs are registered nurses who have a graduate degree in midwifery, meaning they're trained to handle low-risk pregnancies and deliveries. Most CNMs deliver babies in hospitals or birth centers, although some do home births.

In addition to obstetricians and CNMs, **registered nurses (RNs)** attend births to take care of the mother and baby. If you give birth in a teaching hospital, medical students or residents might be present during the birth. Some family doctors also offer prenatal care and deliver babies.

While you're in the hospital, if you choose or if it's necessary for you to receive anesthesia, it will be administered by a trained **anesthesiologist**. A variety of pain-control measures, including pain medication and local, epidural, and general anesthesia, are available in the hospital setting.

Birth Centers

Women who deliver in a birth center are usually those who have already given birth without any problems and whose current pregnancies are considered low risk (meaning they are in good health and are the least likely to develop complications).

Women giving birth to multiples, who have certain medical conditions (such as gestational diabetes or high blood pressure), or whose baby is in the breech position are considered higher risk and should not deliver in a birth center.

Women are carefully screened early in pregnancy and given prenatal care at the birth center to monitor their health throughout their pregnancy.

Natural childbirth is the focus in a birth center. Since epidural anesthesia usually isn't offered, women are free to move around in labor, get in the positions most comfortable to them, spend time in the jacuzzi, etc. Comfort measures (such as hydrotherapy, massage, warm and cold compresses, and visualization and relaxation techniques) are often used. The woman is free to eat and drink as she chooses.

A variety of healthcare professionals operate in the birth center setting. A birth center may employ registered nurses, CNMs, and doulas (professionally trained providers of labor support and/or postpartum care).

Although a doctor is seldom present and medical interventions are rarely done, birth centers may work with a variety of obstetric and pediatric consultants. The professionals affiliated with a birth center work closely together as a team, with the nurse-midwives present and the OB/GYN consultants available if a woman develops a complication during pregnancy or labor that puts her into a higher risk category.

The baby's heart rate is monitored often during labor, typically with a handheld Doppler device. Birth centers do have medical equipment available, such as IV lines and fluids, oxygen for the mother and the infant, and other equipment necessary to treat sick babies and moms.

A birth center can provide natural pain control and pain control with mild narcotic medications, but if a woman decides she wants an epidural, or if complications develop, she must be taken to a hospital.

Birth centers often provide a homey birth experience for the mother, baby, and extended family. In most cases, birth centers are freestanding buildings, although they may be attached to a hospital. Birth centers may be located in residential areas and generally include amenities such as private rooms with soft lighting, showers, and whirlpool tubs. A kitchen may be available for the family to use.

Look for a birth center that is accredited by the Commission for the Accreditation of Birth Centers (CABC). Some states regulate birth centers, so find out if the birth center you choose has all the proper credentials.

Which One Is Right for You?

How do you decide whether a hospital or a birth center is the right choice for you? If you've chosen a particular healthcare provider, he or she may only practice at a particular hospital or birth center, so you should discuss your decision. And check with your health insurance carrier to make sure your choice is covered. In many cases, accredited birth centers as well as hospitals are covered by major insurance companies.

If you have any conditions that classify your pregnancy as higher risk (such as being older than 35, carrying multiple fetuses, or having gestational diabetes or high blood pressure, to name a few), your healthcare provider may advise you to deliver in a hospital where you and your baby can receive medical treatment as necessary. In fact, you might not be eligible to deliver in a birth center because of your risk factors. And if you want interventions such as an epidural or continuous fetal monitoring, a hospital is probably the better choice for you.

For a woman without significant problems in her medical history and whose pregnancy has been classified as low risk, a birth center can be an option. Women who want a natural birth with minimal medical intervention or pain control may feel more comfortable in a birth center, as may those who want friends or family members there for the birthing experience.

Once you've decided on either a hospital or a birth center, you may still have to choose which hospital or which birth center. Before you make a choice, be sure that your healthcare provider—whether he or she is a doctor or a CNM—can deliver at the facilities you're considering.

Also, try to get a tour of the hospital or birth center so you can see for yourself if the staff is friendly and the atmosphere is one in which you'll feel relaxed.

Questions To Ask

Before your labor pains start, get answers to these questions:

If Choosing A Hospital

- Is the hospital easy to get to?

- How is it equipped to handle emergencies?

- What level nursery is available? (Nurseries are rated I, II, or III—a level III neonatal intensive care unit [NICU] is equipped to handle any neonatal emergency. A lower rating may require transportation to a level III NICU.)

- How many deliveries take place at the hospital each year? (A higher number means the hospital has more experience with various birth scenarios.)

- What is the nurse-to-patient ratio? (A ratio of 1:2 is considered good during low-risk labor; a 1:1 ratio is best in complicated cases or during the pushing stage.)

- What are the hospital's statistics for Cesarean sections, episiotomies, and mortality? (Keep in mind, though, that these numbers include high-risk and complicated deliveries.)

- How many labor and support people may be present for the birth?

- What procedures are followed after your baby's birth? Can you breastfeed immediately if desired? Is rooming in available?

- How long is the typical postpartum stay for vaginal deliveries? For C-sections?

- Can the baby and the father stay with you in your room around the clock, if you desire?

If Choosing A Birth Center

- Is the birth center accredited by the Commission for the Accreditation of Birth Centers?

- Is the birth center easy to get to?

- What situations during labor would lead to a transfer to a hospital? How are transfers handled? What emergencies are the transfer facilities able to handle?

- What professionals (such as midwives, doctors, and nurses) are available on staff? On a consulting basis? Are they licensed?

- What childbirth and prenatal education classes are offered?

- What are the center's statistics for hospital transfers, episiotomies, and mortality?

- What procedures are followed after your baby's birth? How long is the typical postpartum stay and how will your baby be examined?

It's wise to choose where to deliver your baby as early in your pregnancy as possible. That way, if complications do arise, you'll be well informed and can concentrate on your health and the health of your baby.

Chapter 49

Labor And Birth

Spot The Signs Of Labor

As you approach your due date, you will be looking for any little sign that labor is about to start. You might notice that your baby has "dropped" or moved lower into your pelvis. This is called "lightening." If you have a pelvic exam during your prenatal visit, your doctor might report changes in your cervix that you cannot feel, but that suggest your body is getting ready. For some women, a flurry of energy and the impulse to cook or clean, called "nesting," is a sign that labor is approaching.

Some signs suggest that labor will begin very soon. Call your doctor or midwife if you have any of the following signs of labor. Call your doctor even if it's weeks before your due date—you might be going into preterm labor. Your doctor or midwife can decide if it's time to go to the hospital or if you should be seen at the office first.

- You have contractions that become stronger at regular and increasingly shorter intervals.

- You have lower back pain and cramping that does not go away.

- Your water breaks (can be a large gush or a continuous trickle).

- You have a bloody (brownish or red-tinged) mucus discharge. This is probably the mucus plug that blocks the cervix. Losing your mucus plug usually means your cervix is dilating (opening up) and becoming thinner and softer (effacing). Labor could start right away or may still be days away.

About This Chapter: This chapter includes text excerpted from "Labor And Birth," Office on Women's Health (OWH), U.S. Department of Health and Human Services (HHS), September 27, 2010. Reviewed March 2017.

Did My Water Break?

It's not always easy to know. If your water breaks, it could be a gush or a slow trickle of amniotic fluid. Rupture of membranes is the medical term for your water breaking. Let your doctor know the time your water breaks and any color or odor. Also, call your doctor if you think your water broke, but are not sure. An easy test can tell your doctor if the leaking fluid is urine (many pregnant women leak urine) or amniotic fluid. Often a woman will go into labor soon after her water breaks. When this doesn't happen, her doctor may want to induce (bring about) labor. This is because once your water breaks, your risk of getting an infection goes up as labor is delayed.

False Labor

Many women, especially first-time mothers-to-be, think they are in labor when they're not. This is called false labor. "Practice" contractions called Braxton Hicks contractions are common in the last weeks of pregnancy or earlier. The tightening of your uterus might startle you. Some might even be painful or take your breath away. It's no wonder that many women mistake Braxton Hicks contractions for the real thing. So don't feel embarrassed if you go to the hospital thinking you're in labor, only to be sent home.

So, how can you tell if your contractions are true labor?

Time them. Use a watch or clock to keep track of the time one contraction starts to the time the next contraction starts, as well as how long each contraction lasts. With true labor, contractions become regular, stronger, and more frequent. Braxton Hicks contractions are not in a regular pattern, and they taper off and go away. Some women find that a change in activity, such as walking or lying down, makes Braxton Hicks contractions go away. This won't happen with true labor. Even with these guidelines, it can be hard to tell if labor is real. *If you ever are unsure if contractions are true labor, call your doctor.*

Stages Of Labor

Labor occurs in three stages. When regular contractions begin, the baby moves down into the pelvis as the cervix both effaces (thins) and dilates (opens). How labor progresses and how long it lasts are different for every woman. But each stage features some milestones that are true for every woman.

First Stage

The first stage begins with the onset of labor and ends when the cervix is fully opened. It is the longest stage of labor, usually lasting about 12 to 19 hours. Many women spend the early part of this first stage at home. You might want to rest, watch TV, hang out with family, or even go for a walk. Most women can drink and eat during labor, which can provide needed energy later. Yet some doctors advise laboring women to avoid solid food as a precaution should a Cesarean delivery be needed. Ask your doctor about eating during labor. While at home, time your contractions and keep your doctor up to date on your progress. Your doctor will tell you when to go to the hospital or birthing center.

At the hospital, your doctor will monitor the progress of your labor by periodically checking your cervix, as well as the baby's position and station (location in the birth canal). Most babies' heads enter the pelvis facing to one side, and then rotate to face down. Sometimes, a baby will be facing up, towards the mother's abdomen. Intense back labor often goes along with this position. Your doctor might try to rotate the baby, or the baby might turn on its own.

As you near the end of the first stage of labor, contractions become longer, stronger, and closer together. Many of the positioning and relaxation tips you learned in childbirth class can help now. Try to find the most comfortable position during contractions and to let your muscles go limp between contractions. Let your support person know how he or she can be helpful, such as by rubbing your lower back, giving you ice chips to suck, or putting a cold washcloth on your forehead.

Sometimes, medicines and other methods are used to help speed up labor that is progressing slowly. Many doctors will rupture the membranes. Although this practice is widely used, studies show that doing so during labor does not help shorten the length of labor.

Your doctor might want to use an electronic fetal monitor to see if blood supply to your baby is okay. For most women, this involves putting two straps around the mother's abdomen. One strap measures the strength and frequency of your contractions. The other strap records how the baby's heartbeat reacts to the contraction.

The most difficult phase of this first stage is the transition. Contractions are very powerful, with very little time to relax in between, as the cervix stretches the last, few centimeters. Many women feel shaky or nauseated. The cervix is fully dilated when it reaches 10 centimeters.

Second Stage

The second stage involves pushing and delivery of your baby. It usually lasts 20 minutes to two hours. You will push hard during contractions, and rest between contractions. Pushing is hard work, and a support person can really help keep you focused. A woman can give birth in many positions, such as squatting, sitting, kneeling, or lying back. Giving birth in an upright position, such as squatting, appears to have some benefits, including shortening this stage of labor and helping to keep the tissue near the birth canal intact. You might find pushing to be easier or more comfortable one way, and you should be allowed to choose the birth position that feels best to you.

When the top of your baby's head fully appears (crowning), your doctor will tell you when to push and deliver your baby. Your doctor may make a small cut, called an episiotomy, to enlarge the vaginal opening. Most women in childbirth do not need episiotomy. Sometimes, forceps (tool shaped like salad-tongs) or suction is used to help guide the baby through the birth canal. This is called assisted vaginal delivery. After your baby is born, the umbilical cord is cut. Make sure to tell your doctor if you or your partner would like to cut the umbilical cord.

Third Stage

The third stage involves delivery of the placenta (afterbirth). It is the shortest stage, lasting five to 30 minutes. Contractions will begin five to 30 minutes after birth, signaling that it's time to deliver the placenta. You might have chills or shakiness. Labor is over once the placenta is delivered. Your doctor will repair the episiotomy and any tears you might have. Now, you can rest and enjoy your newborn!

Managing Labor Pain

Virtually all women worry about how they will cope with the pain of labor and delivery. Childbirth is different for everyone. So no one can predict how you will feel. The amount of pain a woman feels during labor depends partly on the size and position of her baby, the size of her pelvis, her emotions, the strength of the contractions, and her outlook.

Some women do fine with natural methods of pain relief alone. Many women blend natural methods with medications that relieve pain. Building a positive outlook on childbirth and managing fear may also help some women cope with the pain. It is important to realize that labor pain is not like pain due to illness or injury. Instead, it is caused by contractions of the uterus that are pushing your baby down and out of the birth canal. In other words, labor pain has a purpose.

Try the following to help you feel positive about childbirth:

- Take a childbirth class. Call the doctor, midwife, hospital, or birthing center for class information.

- Get information from your doctor or midwife. Write down your questions and talk about them at your regular visits.

- Share your fears and emotions with friends, family, and your partner.

Natural Methods Of Pain Relief

Many natural methods help women to relax and make pain more manageable. Things women do to ease the pain include:

- Trying breathing and relaxation techniques

- Taking warm showers or baths

- Getting massages

- Using heat and cold, such as heat on lower back and cold washcloth on forehead

- Having the supportive care of a loved one, nurse, or doula

- Finding comfortable positions while in labor (stand, crouch, sit, walk, etc.)

- Using a labor ball

- Listening to music

Water And Childbirth

More and more women in the United States are using water to find comfort during labor. This is called *hydrotherapy*. Laboring in a tub of warm water helps women feel physically supported, and keeps them warm and relaxed. Plus, it is easier for laboring women to move and find comfortable positions in the water.

In *waterbirthing*, a woman remains in the water for delivery. The American Academy of Pediatrics (AAP) has expressed concerns about delivering in water because of a lack of studies showing its safety and because of the rare but reported chance of complications. Ask your doctor or midwife if you want to know more about waterbirthing.

Medical Methods Of Pain Relief

While you're in labor, your doctor, midwife, or nurse should ask if you need pain relief. It is her job to help you decide what option is best for you. Nowadays women in labor have many pain relief options that work well and pose small risks when given by a trained and experienced doctor. Doctors also can use different methods for pain relief at different stages of labor. Still, not all options are available at every hospital and birthing center. Plus your health history, allergies, and any problems with your pregnancy will make some methods better than others.

Methods of relieving pain commonly used for labor are described in the Table 49.1 below. Keep in mind that rare, but serious complications sometimes occur. Also, most medicines used

Table 49.1. Methods Of Pain Relief

Method	How It Can Help	Some Disadvantages
Opioids—also called narcotics, are medicines given through a tube inserted in a vein or by injecting the medicine into a muscle. Sometimes, opioids also are given with epidural or spinal blocks.	Opioids can make the pain bearable, and don't affect your ability to push. After getting this kind of pain relief, you can still get an epidural or spinal block later.	• Opioids don't get rid of all the pain, and they are short-acting. • They can make you feel sleepy and drowsy. • They can cause nausea and vomiting. • They can make you feel very itchy. • Opioids cannot be given right before delivery because they may slow the baby's breathing and heart rate at birth.
Epidural and spinal blocks— An epidural involves placing a tube (catheter) into the lower back, into a small space below the spinal cord. Small doses of medicine can be given through the tube as needed throughout labor. With a spinal block, a small dose of medicine is given as a shot into the spinal fluid in the lower back. Spinal blocks usually are given only once during labor.	Epidural and spinal blocks allow most women to be awake and alert with very little pain during labor and childbirth. With epidural, pain relief starts 10 to 20 minutes after the medicine has been given. The degree of numbness you feel can be adjusted throughout your labor. With spinal block, good pain relief starts right away, but it only lasts 1 to 2 hours.	• Although you can move, you might not be able to walk if the medicine used affects motor function. • It can lower your blood pressure, which can slow your baby's heartbeat. Fluids given through IV are given to lower this risk. Fluids can make you shiver. But women in labor often shiver with or without epidural. • If the covering of the spinal chord is punctured, you can get a bad headache. Treatment can help the headache. • Backache for a few days after labor. • Epidural can prolong the first and second stages of labor. If given late in labor or if too much medicine is used, it might be hard to push when the time comes. Studies show that epidural increases risk of assisted vaginal delivery.
Pudendal block—A doctor injects numbing medicine into the vagina and the nearby pudendal nerve. This nerve carries sensation to the lower part of your vagina and vulva.	This is only used late in labor, usually right before the baby's head comes out. With a pudendal block, you have some pain relief but remain awake, alert, and able to push the baby out.	• The baby is not affected by this medicine and it has very few disadvantages.

to manage pain during labor pass freely into the placenta. Ask your doctor how pain relief methods might affect your baby or your ability to breastfeed after delivery.

Inducing Labor

Sometimes, a doctor or midwife might need to induce (bring about) labor. The decision to induce labor often is made when a woman is past her due date but labor has not yet begun or when there is concern about the baby or mother's health. Some specific reasons why labor might be induced include:

- A woman's water has broken (ruptured membranes), but labor has not begun on its own

- Infection inside the uterus

- Baby is growing too slowly

- Complications that arise when the mother's Rh factor is negative and her unborn baby's is positive

- Not enough amniotic fluid

- Complications, such as high blood pressure or preeclampsia

- Health problems in the mother, such as kidney disease or diabetes

The doctor or midwife can use medicines and other methods to open a pregnant woman's cervix, stimulate contractions, and prepare for vaginal birth.

Elective labor induction has become more common in recent years. This is when labor is induced at term but for no medical reason. Some doctors may suggest elective induction due to a woman's discomfort, scheduling issues, or concern that waiting may lead to complications. But the benefits and harms of elective induction are not well understood. For instance, we do not know if elective labor induction leads to higher or lower rates of Cesarean delivery compared to waiting for labor to start on its own. Yet, doctors have ways to assess risk of Cesarean delivery, such as a woman's age, whether it is her first pregnancy, and the status of her cervix. Elective induction (not before 39 weeks) does not appear to affect the health of the baby.

If your doctor suggests inducing labor, talk to your doctor about the possible harms and benefits for both mother and baby, such as the risk of C-section and the risk of low birth weight. You will want to be sure the benefits of inducing labor outweigh the risks of induction and the risks of continuing the pregnancy.

Chapter 50
Having A Doula: Is A Doula For Me?

Having A Doula: Their Benefits And Purpose

The word **doula** is a Greek word meaning women's servant. Women have been serving others in childbirth for many centuries and have proven that support from another woman has a positive impact on the labor process.

What Is A Doula?

A doula is a professional trained in childbirth who provides emotional, physical, and educational support to a mother who is expecting, is experiencing labor, or has recently given birth. The doula's purpose is to help women have a safe, memorable, and empowering birthing experience.

Most often the term *doula* refers to the birth doula, or labor support companion. However, there are also antepartum doulas and postpartum doulas. Most of the following information relates to the labor doula. Doulas can also be referred to as labor companions, labor support specialists, labor support professionals, birth assistants, or labor assistants.

What Does A Doula Do?

Most doula-client relationships begin a few months before the baby is due. During this period, they develop a relationship in which the mother feels free to ask questions, express her fears and concerns, and take an active role in creating a birth plan.

About This Chapter: Text in this chapter is excerpted from "Having A Doula: Is A Doula For Me?" © 2017 American Pregnancy Association. Reprinted with permission.

Most doulas make themselves available to the mother by phone in order to respond to her questions or address any concerns that might arise during the course of the pregnancy. Doulas do not provide any type of medical care. However, they are knowledgeable in many medical aspects of labor and delivery.

As such, they can help their clients gain a better understanding of the procedures and possible complications in late pregnancy or delivery.

During delivery, doulas are in constant and close proximity to the mother. They have the ability to provide comfort with pain-relief techniques including breathing techniques, relaxation techniques, massage, and laboring positions. Doulas also encourage participation from the partner and offer reassurance.

A doula acts as an advocate for the mother, encouraging and helping her fulfill specific desires she might have for her birth. The goal of a doula is to help the mother experience a positive and safe birth, whether an un-medicated birth or a Cesarean.

After the birth, many labor doulas will spend time helping mothers begin the breastfeeding process and encouraging bonding between the new baby and other family members.

What Are The Benefits Of Having A Doula?

Numerous studies have documented the benefits of having a doula present during labor. A recent Cochrane Review, *Continuous Support for Women During Childbirth*, showed a very high number of positive birth outcomes when a doula was present. With the support of a doula, women were less likely to have pain-relief medications administered and less likely to have a Cesarean birth. Women also reported having a more positive childbirth experience.

Other studies have shown that having a doula as a member of the birth team decreases the overall Cesarean rate by 50%, the length of labor by 25%, the use of oxytocin by 40%, and requests for an epidural by 60%.

Doulas often use the power of touch and massage to reduce stress and anxiety during labor. According to physicians Marshal Klaus and John Kennell, massage helps stimulate the production of natural oxytocin. The pituitary gland secretes natural oxytocin to the bloodstream (causing uterine contractions) and to the brain (resulting in feelings of well-being and drowsiness, along with a higher pain threshold).

Historically it was thought that intravenous oxytocin does not cross from the bloodstream to the brain in substantial amounts and, therefore, does not provide the same psychological benefits as natural oxytocin. However, more recent studies indicate that oxytocin administered nasally and/or intravenously may cross from the bloodstream to the brain. Nonetheless, doulas can help mothers experience the benefits of oxytocin naturally without the use of medication.

What About The Father's Role When Using A Doula?

The role of the doula is never to take the place of husbands or partners in labor but rather to compliment and enhance their experience. Today, more husbands play an active role in the birth process. However, some partners prefer to enjoy the delivery without having to stand in as the labor coach.

By having a doula as a part of the birth team, a father is free to do whatever he chooses. Doulas can encourage the father to use comfort techniques and can step in if he wants a break. Having a doula allows the father to support his partner emotionally during labor and birth and to also enjoy the experience without the added pressure of trying to remember everything he learned in childbirth class!.

Are Doulas Only Useful If Planning An Un-Medicated Birth?

The presence of a doula can be beneficial no matter what type of birth you are planning. Many women report needing fewer interventions when they have a doula. But be aware that the primary role of the doula is to help mothers have a safe and pleasant birth–not to help them choose the type of birth.

For women who have decided to have a medicated birth, the doula will provide emotional, informational, and physical support through labor and the administration of medications. Doulas work alongside medicated mothers to help them deal with potential side effects. Doulas may also help with other needs where medication may be inadequate because even with medication, there is likely to be some degree of discomfort.

For a mother facing a Cesarean, a doula can be helpful by providing constant support and encouragement. Often a Cesarean results from an unexpected situation leaving a mother feeling unprepared, disappointed, and lonely. A doula can be attentive to the mother at all times throughout the Cesarean, letting her know what is going on throughout the procedure. This can free the partner to attend to the baby and accompany the newborn to the nursery if there are complications.

What About Other Types Of Doulas?

In addition to labor doulas, there are antepartum doulas and postpartum doulas.

Antepartum doulas provide support to a mother who has been put on bed rest or is experiencing a high risk-pregnancy. They provide informational, emotional, physical, and practical support in circumstances that are often stressful, confusing, and emotionally draining.

Postpartum doulas provide support in the first weeks after birth. They provide informational support about feeding and caring for the baby. They provide physical support by cleaning, cooking meals, and filling in when a new mother needs a break. They provide emotional support by encouraging a mother when she feels overwhelmed.

Some doulas have training in more than one area and are able to serve as more than one type of doula.

Finding A Doula

The key to choosing a doula is to find a person with whom you feel comfortable. Most doulas do not charge for an initial consultation, so take the time to interview as many as necessary until you find a good match.

Questions To Ask A Potential Doula

- What training have you had?

- What services do you provide?

- What are your fees?

- Are you available for my due date?

- What made you decide to become a doula?

- What is your philosophy regarding childbirth?

- Would you be available to meet with me before the birth to discuss my birth plan?

- What happens if for some reason you are not available at the time I give birth?

Chapter 51

Cesarean Birth

Cesarean delivery, also called C-section, is surgery to deliver a baby. The baby is taken out through the mother's abdomen. Most Cesarean births result in healthy babies and mothers. But C-section is major surgery and carries risks. Healing also takes longer than with vaginal birth.

Most healthy pregnant women with no risk factors for problems during labor or delivery have their babies vaginally. Still, the Cesarean birth rate in the United States has risen greatly in recent decades. Today, nearly 1 in 3 women have babies by C-section in this country. The rate was 1 in 5 in 1995.

Public health experts think that many C-sections are unnecessary. So it is important for pregnant women to get the facts about C-sections before they deliver. Women should find out what C-sections are, why they are performed, and the pros and cons of this surgery.

Reasons For C-Sections

Your doctor might recommend a C-section if she or he thinks it is safer for you or your baby than vaginal birth. Some C-sections are planned. But most C-sections are done when unexpected problems happen during delivery. Even so, there are risks of delivering by C-section. Limited studies show that the benefits of having a C-section may outweigh the risks when:

- The mother is carrying more than one baby (twins, triplets, etc.)
- The mother has health problems including HIV infection, herpes infection, and heart disease

About This Chapter: This chapter includes text excerpted from "Labor And Birth," Office on Women's Health (OWH), U.S. Department of Health and Human Services (HHS), September 27, 2010. Reviewed March 2017.

- The mother has dangerously high blood pressure

- The mother has problems with the shape of her pelvis

- There are problems with the placenta

- There are problems with the umbilical cord

- There are problems with the position of the baby, such as breech

- The baby shows signs of distress, such as a slowed heart rate

- The mother has had a previous C-section

Patient-Requested C-Section: Can A Woman Choose?

A growing number of women are asking their doctors for C-sections when there is no medical reason. Some women want a C-section because they fear the pain of childbirth. Others like the convenience of being able to decide when and how to deliver their baby. Still others fear the risks of vaginal delivery including tearing and sexual problems.

But is it safe and ethical for doctors to allow women to choose C-section? The answer is unclear. Only more research on both types of deliveries will provide the answer. In the meantime, many obstetricians feel it is their ethical obligation to talk women out of elective C-sections. Others believe that women should be able to choose a C-section if they understand the risks and benefits.

Experts who believe C-sections should only be performed for medical reasons point to the risks. These include infection, dangerous bleeding, blood transfusions, and blood clots. Babies born by C-section have more breathing problems right after birth. Women who have C-sections stay at the hospital for longer than women who have vaginal births. Plus, recovery from this surgery takes longer and is often more painful than that after a vaginal birth. C-sections also increase the risk of problems in future pregnancies. Women who have had C-sections have a higher risk of uterine rupture. If the uterus ruptures, the life of the baby and mother is in danger.

Supporters of elective C-sections say that this surgery may protect a woman's pelvic organs, reduces the risk of bowel and bladder problems, and is as safe for the baby as vaginal delivery.

The National Institutes of Health (NIH) and American College of Obstetricians (ACOG) agree that a doctor's decision to perform a C-section at the request of a patient should be made on a case-by-case basis and be consistent with ethical principles. ACOG states that "if the physician believes that (Cesarean) delivery promotes the overall health and welfare of the woman and her fetus more than vaginal birth, he or she is ethically justified in performing" a C-section. Both organizations also say that C-section should never be scheduled before a pregnancy is 39 weeks, or the lungs are mature, unless there is medical need.

The C-Section Experience

Most C-sections are unplanned. So, learning about C-sections is important for all women who are pregnant. Whether a C-section is planned or comes up during labor, it can be a positive birth experience for many women. The overview that follows will help you to know what to expect during a nonemergency C-section and what questions to ask

Before Surgery

Cesarean delivery takes about 45 to 60 minutes. It takes place in an operating room. So if you were in a labor and delivery room, you will be moved to an operating room. Often, the mood of the operating room is unhurried and relaxed. A doctor will give you medicine through an epidural or spinal block, which will block the feeling of pain in part of your body but allow you to stay awake and alert. The spinal block works right away and completely numbs your body from the chest down. The epidural takes away pain, but you might be aware of some tugging or pushing. Medicine that makes you fall asleep and lose all awareness is usually only used in emergency situations. Your abdomen will be cleaned and prepped. You will have an IV for fluids and medicines. A nurse will insert a catheter to drain urine from your bladder. This is to protect the bladder from harm during surgery. Your heart rate, blood pressure, and breathing also will be monitored. Questions to ask:

- Can I have a support person with me during the operation?

- What are my options for blocking pain?

- Can I have music played during the surgery?

- Will I be able to watch the surgery if I want?

During Surgery

The doctor will make two incisions. The first is about 6 inches long and goes through the skin, fat, and muscle. Most incisions are made side to side and low on the abdomen, called a bikini incision. Next, the doctor will make an incision to open the uterus. The opening is made just wide enough for the baby to fit through. One doctor will use a hand to support the baby while another doctor pushes the uterus to help push that baby out. Fluid will be suctioned out of your baby's mouth and nose. The doctor will hold up your baby for you to see. Once your baby is delivered, the umbilical cord is cut, and the placenta is removed. Then, the doctor cleans and stitches up the uterus and abdomen. The repair takes up most of the surgery time. Questions to ask:

- Can my partner cut the umbilical cord?

- What happens to my baby right after delivery?

- Can I hold and touch my baby during the surgery repair?

- When is it okay for me to try to breastfeed?

- When can my partner take pictures or video?

After Surgery

You will be moved to a recovery room and monitored for a few hours. You might feel shaky, nauseated, and very sleepy. Later, you will be brought to a hospital room. When you and your baby are ready, you can hold, snuggle, and nurse your baby. Many people will be excited to see you. But don't accept too many visitors. Use your time in the hospital, usually about four days, to rest and bond with your baby. C-section is major surgery, and recovery takes about six weeks (not counting the fatigue of new motherhood). In the weeks ahead, you will need to focus on healing, getting as much rest as possible, and bonding with your baby—nothing else. Be careful about taking on too much and accept help as needed. Questions to ask:

- Can my baby be brought to me in the recovery room?

- What are the best positions for me to breastfeed?

Vaginal Birth After C-Section (VBAC)?

Some women who have delivered previous babies by C-section would like to have their next baby vaginally. This is called vaginal delivery after C-section or VBAC. Women give many reasons for wanting a VBAC. Some want to avoid the risks and long recovery of surgery. Others want to experience vaginal delivery.

Today, VBAC is a reasonable and safe choice for most women with prior Cesarean delivery, including some women who have had more than one Cesarean delivery.

Chapter 52
Recovering From Childbirth

Right now, you are focused on caring for your new baby. But new mothers must take special care of their bodies after giving birth and while breastfeeding, too. Doing so will help you to regain your energy and strength. When you take care of yourself, you are able to best care for and enjoy your baby.

Getting Rest

The first few days at home after having your baby are a time for rest and recovery—physically and emotionally. You need to focus your energy on yourself and on getting to know your new baby. Even though you may be very excited and have requests for lots of visits from family and friends, try to limit visitors and get as much rest as possible. Don't expect to keep your house perfect. You may find that all you can do is eat, sleep, and care for your baby. And that is perfectly okay. Learn to pace yourself from the first day that you arrive back home. Try to lie down or nap while the baby naps. Don't try to do too much around the house. Allow others to help you and don't be afraid to ask for help with cleaning, laundry, meals, or with caring for the baby.

Physical Changes

After the birth of your baby, your doctor will talk with you about things you will experience as your body starts to recover.

- You will have vaginal discharge called lochia. It is the tissue and blood that lined your uterus during pregnancy. It is heavy and bright red at first, becoming lighter in flow and color until it goes aware after a few weeks.

About This Chapter: This chapter includes text excerpted from "Recovering From Birth," Office on Women's Health (OWH), U.S. Department of Health and Human Services (HHS), September 27, 2010. Reviewed March 2017.

- You might also have swelling in your legs and feet. You can reduce swelling by keeping your feet elevated when possible.

- You might feel constipated. Try to drink plenty of water and eat fresh fruits and vegetables.

- Menstrual-like cramping is common, especially if you are breastfeeding. Your breast milk will come in within three to six days after your delivery. Even if you are not breastfeeding, you can have milk leaking from your nipples, and your breasts might feel full, tender, or uncomfortable.

- Follow your doctor's instructions on how much activity, like climbing stairs or walking, you can do for the next few weeks.

Your doctor will check your recovery at your postpartum visit, about six weeks after birth. Ask about resuming normal activities, as well as eating and fitness plans to help you return to a healthy weight. Also ask your doctor about having sex and birth control. Your period could return in six to eight weeks, or sooner if you do not breastfeed. If you breastfeed, your period might not resume for many months. Still, using reliable birth control is the best way to prevent pregnancy until you want to have another baby.

Some women develop thyroid problems in the first year after giving birth. This is called postpartum thyroiditis. It often begins with overactive thyroid, which lasts two to four months. Most women then develop symptoms of an underactive thyroid, which can last up to a year. Thyroid problems are easy to overlook as many symptoms, such as fatigue, sleep problems, low energy, and changes in weight, are common after having a baby. Talk to your doctor if you have symptoms that do not go away. An underactive thyroid needs to be treated. In most cases, thyroid function returns to normal as the thyroid heals. But some women develop permanent underactive thyroid disease, called Hashimoto disease, and need lifelong treatment.

Regaining A Healthy Weight And Shape

Both pregnancy and labor can affect a woman's body. After giving birth, you will lose about 10 pounds right away and a little more as body fluid levels decrease. Don't expect or try to lose additional pregnancy weight right away. Gradual weight loss over several months is the safest way, especially if you are breastfeeding. Nursing mothers can safely lose a moderate amount of weight without affecting their milk supply or their babies' growth.

A healthy eating plan along with regular physical fitness might be all you need to return to a healthy weight. If you are not losing weight or losing weight too slowly, cut back on foods with added sugars and fats, like soft drinks, desserts, fried foods, fatty meats, and alcohol. Keep in mind, nursing mothers should avoid alcohol. By cutting back on "extras," you can focus on healthy, well-balanced food choices that will keep your energy level up and help you get the nutrients you and your baby need for good health. Make sure to talk to your doctor before you start any type of diet or exercise plan.

Returning to a healthy weight after you deliver your baby may lower your chances of diabetes, heart disease, and other weight-related problems.

Wait until your six-week checkup before trying to slim down. If you are breastfeeding, wait until your baby is at least two months old. By cutting about 500 calories a day from your diet, you can lose about a pound and a half a week.

Breastfeeding may make it easier for you to lose weight because your body burns extra energy to produce milk. Your calorie needs when breastfeeding depend on how much body fat you have and how active you are.

(Source: "Healthy Weight Management For New Moms," Smokefree Women, U.S. Department of Health and Human Services (HHS).)

Feeling Blue

After childbirth you may feel sad, weepy, and overwhelmed for a few days. Many new mothers have the "baby blues" after giving birth. Changing hormones, anxiety about caring for the baby, and lack of sleep all affect your emotions.

Be patient with yourself. These feelings are normal and usually go away quickly. But if sadness lasts more than two weeks, go see your doctor. Don't wait until you postpartum visit to do so. You might have a serious but treatable condition called postpartum depression. Postpartum depression can happen any time within the first year after birth.

Signs of postpartum depression include:

- Feeling restless or irritable

- Feeling sad, depressed, or crying a lot

- Having no energy

- Having headaches, chest pains, heart palpitations (the heart being fast and feeling like it is skipping beats), numbness, or hyperventilation (fast and shallow breathing)

- Not being able to sleep, being very tired, or both

- Not being able to eat and weight loss

- Overeating and weight gain

- Trouble focusing, remembering, or making decisions

- Being overly worried about the baby

- Not having any interest in the baby

- Feeling worthless and guilty

- Having no interest or getting no pleasure from activities like sex and socializing

- Thoughts of harming your baby or yourself

Some women don't tell anyone about their symptoms because they feel embarrassed or guilty about having these feelings at a time when they think they should be happy. Don't let this happen to you! Postpartum depression can make it hard to take care of your baby. Infants with mothers with postpartum depression can have delays in learning how to talk. They can have problems with emotional bonding. Your doctor can help you feel better and get back to enjoying your new baby. Therapy and/or medicine can treat postpartum depression.

Emerging research suggests that 1 in 10 new fathers may experience depression during or after pregnancy. Although more research is needed, having depression may make it harder to be a good father and perhaps affect the baby's development. Having depression may also be related to a mother's depression. Expecting or new fathers with emotional problems or symptoms of depression should talk to their doctors. Depression is a treatable illness.

Part Six
Your Newborn

Chapter 53

Your Baby's First Hours Of Life

After months of waiting, finally, your new baby has arrived! Mothers-to-be often spend so much time in anticipation of labor, they don't think about or even know what to expect during the first hours after delivery.

What Newborns Look Like

You might be surprised by how your newborn looks at birth. If you had a vaginal delivery, your baby entered this world through a narrow and boney passage. It's not uncommon for newborns to be born bluish, bruised, and with a misshapen head. An ear might be folded over. Your baby may have a complete head of hair or be bald. Your baby also will have a thick, pasty, whitish coating, which protected the skin in the womb. This will wash away during the first bathing.

Once your baby is placed into your arms, your gaze will go right to his or her eyes. Most newborns open their eyes soon after birth. Eyes will be brown or bluish-gray at first. Looking over your baby, you might notice that the face is a little puffy. You might notice small white bumps inside your baby's mouth or on his or her tongue. Your baby might be very wrinkly. Some babies, especially those born early, are covered in soft, fine hair, which will come off in a couple of weeks. Your baby's skin might have various colored marks, blotches, or rashes, and fingernails could be long. You might also notice that your baby's breasts and penis or vulva are a bit swollen.

About This Chapter: This chapter includes text excerpted from "Your Baby's First Hours Of Life," Office on Women's Health (OWH), U.S. Department of Health and Human Services (HHS), September 27, 2010. Reviewed March 2017.

How your baby looks will change from day to day, and many of the early marks of childbirth go away with time. If you have any concerns about something you see, talk to your doctor. After a few weeks, your newborn will look more and more like the baby you pictured in your dreams.

Bonding With Your Baby

Spending time with your baby in those first hours of life is very special. Although you might be tired, your newborn could be quite alert after birth. Cuddle your baby skin-to-skin. Let your baby get to know your voice and study your face. Your baby can see up to about two feet away. You might notice that your baby throws his or her arms out if someone turns on a light or makes a sudden noise. This is called the startle response. Babies also are born with grasp and sucking reflexes. Put your finger in your baby's palm and watch how she or he knows to squeeze it. Feed your baby when she or he shows signs of hunger.

Medical Care For Your Newborn

Right after birth, babies need many important tests and procedures to ensure their health. Some of these are even required by law. But as long as the baby is healthy, everything but the Apgar test can wait for at least an hour. Delaying further medical care will preserve the precious first moments of life for you, your partner, and the baby. A baby who has not been poked and prodded may be more willing to nurse and cuddle. So before delivery, talk to your doctor or midwife about delaying shots, medicine, and tests. At the same time, please don't assume "everything is being taken care of." As a parent, it's your job to make sure your newborn gets all the necessary and appropriate vaccines and tests in a timely manner.

The following tests and procedures are recommended or required in most hospitals in the United States:

Apgar Evaluation

The Apgar test is a quick way for doctors to figure out if the baby is healthy or needs extra medical care. Apgar tests are usually done twice: one minute after birth and again five minutes after birth. Doctors and nurses measure five signs of the baby's condition. These are:

- Heart rate

- Breathing

- Activity and muscle tone

- Reflexes

- Skin color

Apgar scores range from zero to 10. A baby who scores seven or more is considered very healthy. But a lower score doesn't always mean there is something wrong. Perfectly healthy babies often have low Apgar scores in the first minute of life.

In more than 98 percent of cases, the Apgar score reaches seven after five minutes of life. When it does not, the baby needs medical care and close monitoring.

Eye Care

Your baby may receive eye drops or ointment to prevent eye infections they can get during delivery. Sexually transmitted infections (STIs), including gonorrhea and chlamydia, are a main cause of newborn eye infections. These infections can cause blindness if not treated.

Medicines used can sting and/or blur the baby's vision. So you may want to postpone this treatment for a little while.

Some parents question whether this treatment is really necessary. Many women at low risk for STIs do not want their newborns to receive eye medicine. But there is no evidence to suggest that this medicine harms the baby.

It is important to note that even pregnant women who test negative for STIs may get an infection by the time of delivery. Plus, most women with gonorrhea and/or chlamydia don't know it because they have no symptoms.

Vitamin K Shot

The American Academy of Pediatrics (AAP) recommends that all newborns receive a shot of vitamin K in the upper leg. Newborns usually have low levels of vitamin K in their bodies. This vitamin is needed for the blood to clot. Low levels of vitamin K can cause a rare but serious bleeding problem. Research shows that vitamin K shots prevent dangerous bleeding in newborns.

Newborns probably feel pain when the shot is given. But afterwards babies don't seem to have any discomfort. Since it may be uncomfortable for the baby, you may want to postpone this shot for a little while.

Newborn Metabolic Screening

Doctors or nurses prick your baby's heel to take a tiny sample of blood. They use this blood to test for many diseases. All babies should be tested because a few babies may look healthy but have a rare health problem. A blood test is the only way to find out about these problems. If found right away, serious problems like developmental disabilities, organ damage, blindness, and even death might be prevented.

All 50 states and U.S. territories screen newborns for phenylketonuria (PKU), hypothyroidism, galactosemia, and sickle cell disease. But many states routinely test for up to 30 different diseases. The March of Dimes recommends that all newborns be tested for at least 29 diseases.

You can find out what tests are offered in your state by contacting your state's health department or newborn screening program.

Hearing Test

Most babies have a hearing screening soon after birth, usually before they leave the hospital. Tiny earphones or microphones are used to see how the baby reacts to sounds. All newborns need a hearing screening because hearing defects are not uncommon and hearing loss can be hard to detect in babies and young children. When problems are found early, children can get the services they need at an early age. This might prevent delays in speech, language, and thinking. Ask your hospital or your baby's doctor about newborn hearing screening.

Hepatitis B Vaccine

All newborns should get a vaccine to protect against the hepatitis B virus (HBV) before leaving the hospital. Sadly, 1 in 5 babies at risk of HBV infection leaves the hospital without receiving the vaccine and treatment shown to protect newborns, even if exposed to HBV at birth. HBV can cause a lifelong infection, serious liver damage, and even death.

The hepatitis B vaccine (HepB) is a series of three different shots. The American Academy of Pediatrics (AAP) and the Centers for Disease Control and Prevention (CDC) recommend that all newborns get the first HepB shot before leaving the hospital. If the mother has HBV, her baby should also get a Hepatitis B immune globulin (HBIG) shot within 12 hours of birth. The second HepB shot should be given one to two months after birth. The third HepB shot should be given no earlier than 24 weeks of age, but before 18 months of age.

Complete Checkup

Soon after delivery most doctors or nurses also:

- Measure the newborn's weight, length, and head.

- Take the baby's temperature.

- Measure that baby's breathing and heart rate.

- Give the baby a bath and clean the umbilical cord stump.

Chapter 54

Breastfeeding

Every woman's journey to motherhood is different, but one of the first decisions a new mom makes is how to feed her child.

When you choose to breastfeed, you make an investment in your baby's future. Breastfeeding allows you to make the food that is perfect for your baby. Your milk gives your baby the healthy start that will last a lifetime.

Breastfeeding also:

- Protects your baby

- Benefits your health

- May make your life easier

- Benefits society

What Is Colostrum And How Does It Help My Baby?

Your breastmilk helps your baby grow healthy and strong from day one.

- **Your first milk is liquid gold.** Called liquid gold for its deep yellow color, colostrum is the thick first milk that you make during pregnancy and just after birth. This milk is very rich in nutrients and includes antibodies to protect your baby from infections. Colostrum also helps your newborn infant's digestive system to grow and function. Your baby

About This Chapter: This chapter includes text excerpted from "Why Breastfeeding Is Important," Office on Women's Health (OWH), U.S. Department of Health and Human Services (HHS), July 21, 2014.

gets only a small amount of colostrum at each feeding, because the stomach of a new-born infant is tiny and can hold only a small amount.

- **Your milk changes as your baby grows.** Colostrum changes into mature milk by the third to fifth day after birth. This mature milk has just the right amount of fat, sugar, water, and protein to help your baby continue to grow. It looks thinner than colostrum, but it has the nutrients and antibodies your baby needs for healthy growth.

What Health Benefits Does Breastfeeding Give My Baby?

The cells, hormones, and antibodies in breastmilk protect babies from illness. This protection is unique and changes to meet your baby's needs.

Research suggests that breastfed babies have lower risks of:

- Asthma
- Childhood leukemia
- Childhood obesity
- Ear infections
- Eczema (atopic dermatitis)
- Diarrhea and vomiting
- Lower respiratory infections
- Necrotizing enterocolitis, a disease that affects the gastrointestinal tract in preterm infants
- Sudden infant death syndrome (SIDS)
- Type 2 diabetes

Does My Breastfeeding Baby Need More Vitamin D?

Maybe. Vitamin D is needed to build strong bones. All infants and children should get at least 400 International Units (IU) of vitamin D each day.

To meet this need, your child's doctor may recommend that you give your baby a vitamin D supplement of 400 IU each day. This should start in the first few days of life. You can buy vitamin D supplements for infants at a drugstore or grocery store.

Even though sunlight is a major source of vitamin D, it is hard to measure how much sunlight your baby gets and sun exposure can be harmful. Once your baby is weaned from breastmilk, talk to your baby's doctor about whether your baby still needs vitamin D supplements. Some children do not get enough vitamin D from the food they eat.

What Are The Health Benefits Of Breastfeeding For Mothers?

Breastfeeding helps a mother's health and healing following childbirth. Breastfeeding leads to a lower risk of these health problems in mothers:

- Type 2 diabetes
- Certain types of breast cancer
- Ovarian cancer

How Does Breastfeeding Compare To Formula-feeding?

- **Formula can be harder for your baby to digest.** For most babies, especially premature babies, breastmilk substitutes like formula are harder to digest than breastmilk. Formula is made from cow's milk, and it often takes time for babies' stomachs to adjust to digesting it.

- **Life can be easier for you when you breastfeed.** Breastfeeding may seem like it takes a little more effort than formula-feeding at first. But breastfeeding can make your life easier once you and your baby settle into a good routine. When you breastfeed, there are no bottles and nipples to sterilize. You do not have to buy, measure, and mix formula. And there are no bottles to warm in the middle of the night! When you breastfeed, you can satisfy your baby's hunger right away.

- **Not breastfeeding costs money.** Formula and feeding supplies can cost well over $1,500 each year. Breastfed babies may also be sick less often, which can help keep your baby's health costs lower.

- **Breastfeeding keeps mother and baby close.** Physical contact is important to newborns. It helps them feel more secure, warm, and comforted. Mothers also benefit from this closeness. The skin-to-skin contact boosts your oxytocin levels. Oxytocin is a hormone that helps breastmilk flow and can calm the mother.

> **Did You Know?**
>
> In some situations, formula-feeding can save lives.
>
> - Very rarely, babies are born unable to tolerate milk of any kind. These babies must have an infant formula that is hypoallergenic, dairy free, or lactose free. A wide selection of specialist baby formulas now on the market include soy formula, hydrolyzed formula, lactose-free formula, and hypoallergenic formula.
> - Your baby may need formula if you have certain health conditions that won't allow you to breastfeed and you do not have access to donor breast milk.
>
> Talk to your doctor before feeding your baby anything besides your breastmilk.

Can Breastfeeding Help Me Lose Weight?

Besides giving your baby nourishment and helping to keep your baby from becoming sick, breastfeeding may help you lose weight. Many women who breastfed their babies said it helped them get back to their pre-pregnancy weight more quickly, but experts are still looking at the effects of breastfeeding on weight loss.

How Does Breastfeeding Benefit Society?

Society benefits overall when mothers breastfeed.

- **Breastfeeding saves lives.** Recent research shows that if 90 percent of families breastfed exclusively for 6 months, nearly 1,000 deaths among infants could be prevented.

- **Breastfeeding saves money.** The United States would also save $2.2 billion per year—medical care costs are lower for fully breastfed infants than never-breastfed infants. Breastfed infants usually need fewer sick care visits, prescriptions, and hospitalizations.

- **Breastfeeding also helps make a more productive workforce.** Mothers who breastfeed miss less work to care for sick infants than mothers who feed their infants formula. Employer medical costs are also lower.

- **Breastfeeding is better for the environment.** Formula cans and bottle supplies create more trash and plastic waste. Your milk is a renewable resource that comes packaged and warmed.

How Does Breastfeeding Help In An Emergency?

During an emergency, such as natural disaster, breastfeeding can save your baby's life:

- Breastfeeding protects your baby from the risks of an unclean water supply.

- Breastfeeding can help protect your baby against respiratory illnesses and diarrhea.

- Your milk is always at the right temperature for your baby. It helps to keep your baby's body temperature from dropping too low.

- Your milk is readily available without needing other supplies.

Chapter 55
Bringing Your Baby Home

Whether your baby comes home from the hospital right away, arrives later (perhaps after a stay in the neonatal intensive care unit), or comes through an adoption agency, the homecoming of your little one is a major event you've probably often imagined. Here's how to be prepared.

Leaving The Hospital

Moms-to-be sometimes pack clothes for the trip home before even going to the hospital—or they may wait to see what the weather brings and have their partner bring clothing for both themselves and the baby. Plan to bring loose-fitting clothing for yourself with a drawstring or elastic waist because you most likely won't fit into your pre-pregnancy outfits yet.

Babies are often overdressed for the first trip home. Dress your baby as you would dress yourself. So, if you'd be too warm in a knitted hat during the summer, your baby probably will be, too.

In warm weather, dress your baby in a T-shirt and light cotton pants or a baby blanket over bare legs. If it's cold, put footie pajamas, a hat, and warm blanket over your baby. But be sure to keep all blankets far from your baby's face to avoid suffocation.

Chances are much better that you'll bring home a calm, contented baby if you don't spend a lot of time at the hospital trying to dress your newborn in a complicated outfit that requires pushing and pulling your baby's arms and legs.

About This Chapter: Text in this chapter is © 1995-2017. The Nemour Foundation/KidsHealth®. Reprinted with permission.

If you haven't already made the arrangements with your baby's healthcare provider, make sure to ask when the baby's first checkup should be scheduled before you leave the hospital. Depending on the circumstances, some premature babies also go home with a special monitor for checking breathing and heart rate, and you may be taught infant cardiopulmonary resuscitation (CPR).

But whether your baby is full-term or premature, don't feel rushed out the door—have your questions answered before you leave the hospital. And if you find yourself wondering about anything—from bathing to breastfeeding to burping—ask your nurse, lactation consultant, or your baby's doctor.

The Car Trip

The most important item for the trip home is a proper child safety seat (car seat). Every state requires parents to have one before leaving the hospital because it's one of the best ways to protect your baby.

Even for a short trip, it's never safe for one of you to hold your baby in your arms while the other drives. Your baby could be pulled from your arms and thrown against the dashboard by a quick stop.

Consider buying, renting, or borrowing a car seat before your baby's born, when you have time to choose carefully. There are two kinds of car seats for babies: infant-only seats (which must be replaced when your baby weighs 22 to 35 pounds, depending on the type of seat) and convertible seats that accommodate both infants and older children.

Infant-only seats are designed for rear-facing use only and fit infants better than convertible seats. The American Academy of Pediatrics (AAP) recommends that infants and toddlers ride in a rear-facing seat until they are 2 years old or until they have reached the maximum weight and height limits recommended by the manufacturer. (If your baby exceeds the weight recommended by the manufacturer before the second birthday, you'll need to use a convertible seat designed for bigger babies.)

Some parents of newborns find that a "travel system" (which includes a stroller and an infant-only car seat that can be attached to the stroller) makes it much smoother to transition babies—especially sleeping ones—from the car to the stroller.

Convertible seats face toward the rear until your baby is at least 2 years old or has reached the maximum weight and height limits recommended by the manufacturer. A child who reaches the height and weight limits before age 2 is safest in a bigger convertible seat and kept rear facing. Kids who are small can remain in rear-facing seats even after age 2. (Follow the manufacturer's guidelines for when to turn the seat.)

Never put a rear-facing infant or convertible seat in the front seat of your car—always use the rear seat. Passenger-side airbags in the front seat cabin are hazardous for both rear- and forward-facing car seats, and most accidents happen at the front passenger area of the car. When it's cold, strap your baby in snugly first, then put blankets over the baby.

If you borrow a car seat, make sure that it's not more than 6 years old and was never in a crash (even if it looks OK, it could be structurally unsound). Avoid seats that are missing parts or aren't labeled with the manufacture date and model number (you'll have no way to know about recalls).

Also, check the seat for the manufacturer's recommended "expiration date." If you have any doubts about the seat's history, or if it's cracked or shows signs of wear and tear, don't use it.

Ask at your prenatal classes, healthcare provider's office, hospital, or insurance company about rental or loan programs for car seats—they're quite common.

When buying a new seat, it's important to remember that there isn't one type of seat that's safest or best; get one that fits and can be correctly installed in your car. And higher price doesn't necessarily indicate a seat's quality—it could simply mean the seat has added features that you may or may not want or use. Also, be sure to register your new seat so you can be notified of any problems or recalls.

The most common problem involving car seats is improper installation (according to the National Highway Traffic Safety Administration (NHTSA), the majority of all car seats are installed incorrectly). Recently, LATCH (Lower Anchors and Tethers for Children) car seats have become standard in the United States, but a large percentage of these seats are improperly installed too.

Don't trust illustrations or store displays. Follow the manufacturer's instructions (and keep them handy). Ask your doctor or nurse about local resources where your car seat can be checked by someone specifically trained to evaluate car seat installations. Many hospitals, police and fire stations, and even car dealerships offer this type of service for free. Make sure that the evaluation is done by someone trained and experienced.

If you're bringing your baby home from the intensive care unit, bring the car seat to the hospital ahead of time, so the staff can see if it will work for your baby. If special health concerns rule out a standard restraint, ask your child's doctor to recommend car seats for children with special needs.

First-Time Feelings

Don't be surprised if you have mixed emotions as you bring your baby home, especially if this is your first child. You'll likely be nervous. In fact, you may actually feel terrified as you realize that you've given up a certain amount of control over your life.

If your baby wasn't with you much at the hospital, you may not know what sort of schedule your little bundle of joy will keep. But you'll know before long—although babies' schedules do change a lot during those early months. You'll be less stressed if you don't overschedule yourself and can go with the flow.

Depending upon your labor and delivery experience, you may feel physically drained and sore. Your hormones may be struggling to catch up, too. Meanwhile, your partner may feel a little left out if you're totally engrossed with the baby.

You might have other kids awaiting the arrival of this newest family member. Or you may be dealing with a pet who's wondering what's suddenly drawn everyone's attention. And the expectations of new grandparents, competitive siblings, or friends can also make the home-coming stressful.

Your baby's first extended crying period at home will be difficult. Remember: young babies typically cry for 1 to 5 hours within a 24-hour period, and can't always be calmed. Crying usually decreases gradually after the first several weeks. Although it may seem impossible now, in a few months it will be difficult to recall your baby's seemingly endless crying episodes.

The Home Front

Introducing your baby to others at home can be challenging. If you have other kids, be sure to spend some quality time with each of them. Some parents bring home gifts from the new baby for big brothers and sisters. At first, you can expect some jealousy, especially if the main focus of your attention for several years suddenly has new competition. Encourage siblings to "help" you care for this newest family member.

If you have a pet, ask your partner to bring home a blanket with the baby's scent on it and place it near the pet—even before leaving the hospital. Then, when you come home, the pet will already be somewhat familiar with the baby. But remember to never leave pets alone with newborns.

Family And Friends

Ask your partner to be the gatekeeper for visitors and to limit the number of guests at first. You'll be glad later on if you take some time now to rest and become comfortable with your new situation. Although babies typically aren't shy around strangers for the first 3 months or so, they may become overstimulated and tired if too many people are around.

If you have voice mail or a telephone answering machine, consider changing your message to give the vital statistics of your new arrival. You might say something like: "Our newest family member has arrived. Her name is Julia Marie; she was born on Tuesday, and weighed 7 pounds, 10 ounces. We're all fine and adjusting to our new life. If you'd like us to call you back when it's convenient, please leave your name and number."

Don't be shy about accepting visitors slowly. Ask anyone who's ill to wait until they're feeling well and no longer contagious before they visit. You shouldn't hesitate to ask visitors to wash their hands before holding your baby because a newborn baby's immune system is not fully developed.

When To Call The Doctor

Your baby's healthcare provider expects calls from new parents on many topics, including breastfeeding and health concerns. They'd rather have you call than worry about something needlessly.

If you wonder whether you should call the doctor's office, do it, especially if you see something unexpected or different that concerns you. Call if you see any of these signs:

- rectal temperature of 100.4°F (38°C) or higher (in babies younger than 2 months)
- symptoms of dehydration (crying without tears, sunken eyes, a depression in the soft spot on baby's head, no wet diapers in 6 to 8 hours)
- a soft spot that bulges when your baby's quiet and upright
- a baby that is difficult to rouse
- rapid or labored breathing (call 911 if your baby has breathing difficulty and begins turning bluish around the lips or mouth)
- repeated forceful vomiting or an inability to keep fluids down
- bloody vomit or stool
- more than eight diarrhea stools in 8 hours

If your concern is urgent, call your doctor and take your child to the emergency room. Remember, with young infants, minor conditions can sometimes change quickly.

Chapter 56
Newborn Care And Safety

If this is your first baby, you might worry that you are not ready to take care of a newborn. You're not alone. Lots of new parents feel unprepared when it's time to bring their new babies home from the hospital. You can take steps to help yourself get ready for the transition home.

Newborn Care

Taking a newborn care class during your pregnancy can prepare you for the real thing. But feeding and diapering a baby doll isn't quite the same. During your hospital stay, make sure to ask the nurses for help with basic baby care. Don't hesitate to ask the nurse to show you how to do something more than once! Remember, practice makes perfect. Before discharge, make sure you—and your partner—are comfortable with these newborn care basics:

- Handling a newborn, including supporting your baby's neck
- Changing your baby's diaper
- Bathing your baby
- Dressing your baby
- Swaddling your baby
- Feeding and burping your baby
- Cleaning the umbilical cord

About This Chapter: This chapter includes text excerpted from "Newborn Care And Safety," Office on Women's Health (OWH), U.S. Department of Health and Human Services (HHS), September 27, 2010. Reviewed March 2017.

- Caring for a healing circumcision

- Using a bulb syringe to clear your baby's nasal passages

- Taking a newborn's temperature

- Tips for soothing your baby

Before leaving the hospital, ask about home visits by a nurse or healthcare worker. Many new parents appreciate somebody checking in with them and their baby a few days after coming home. If you are breastfeeding, ask whether a lactation consultant can come to your home to provide follow-up support, as well as other resources in your community, such as peer support groups.

Many first-time parents also welcome the help of a family member or friend who has "been there." Having a support person stay with you for a few days can give you the confidence to go at it alone in the weeks ahead. Try to arrange this before delivery.

Your baby's first doctor's visit is another good time to ask about any infant care questions you might have. Ask about reasons to call the doctor. Also ask about what vaccines your baby needs and when. Infants and young children need vaccines because the diseases they protect against can strike at an early age and can be very dangerous in childhood. This includes rare diseases and more common ones, such as the flu.

Sudden Infant Death Syndrome (SIDS)

Since 1992, the American Academy of Pediatrics (AAP) has recommended that infants be placed to sleep on their backs to reduce the risk of sudden infant death syndrome (SIDS), also called crib death. SIDS is the sudden and unexplained death of a baby under 1 year of age. Even though there is no way to know which babies might die of SIDS, there are some things that you can do to make your baby safer:

- Always place your baby on his or her back to sleep, even for naps. This is the safest sleep position for a healthy baby to reduce the risk of SIDS.

- Place your baby on a firm mattress, such as in a safety-approved crib. Research has shown that placing a baby to sleep on soft mattresses, sofas, sofa cushions, waterbeds, sheepskins, or other soft surfaces raises the risk of SIDS.

- Remove soft, fluffy, and loose bedding and stuffed toys from your baby's sleep area. Make sure you keep all pillows, quilts, stuffed toys, and other soft items away from your baby's sleep area.

- Do not use infant sleep positioners. Using a positioner to hold an infant on his or her back or side for sleep is dangerous and not needed.

- Make sure everyone who cares for your baby knows to place your baby on his or her back to sleep and about the dangers of soft bedding. Talk to child care providers, grandparents, babysitters, and all caregivers about SIDS risk. Remember, every sleep time counts.

- Make sure your baby's face and head stay uncovered during sleep. Keep blankets and other coverings away from your baby's mouth and nose. The best way to do this is to dress the baby in sleep clothing so you will not have to use any other covering over the baby. If you do use a blanket or another covering, make sure that the baby's feet are at the bottom of the crib, the blanket is no higher than the baby's chest, and the blanket is tucked in around the bottom of the crib mattress.

- Do not allow smoking around your baby. Don't smoke before or after the birth of your baby and make sure no one smokes around your baby.

- Don't let your baby get too warm during sleep. Keep your baby warm during sleep, but not too warm. Your baby's room should be at a temperature that is comfortable for an adult. Too many layers of clothing or blankets can overheat your baby.

Some mothers worry if the baby rolls over during the night. However, by the time your baby is able to roll over by herself, the risk for SIDS is much lower. During the time of greatest risk, 2 to 4 months of age, most babies are not able to turn over from their backs to their stomachs.

Part Seven
Teen Parenting Problems And Solutions

Chapter 57
Completing Your Education

Although the rate of teenage pregnancy in the United States has been in steady decline for many years, having dropped 64 percent since a peak in 1991, it's still one of the highest among western industrialized nations. The result, according to the Centers for Disease Control and Prevention (CDC), is that around 250,000 babies are born to mothers aged 15–19 each year. And teenage mothers face many unique challenges, including health issues, economic hardship, social interactions, and family and relationship difficulties. Another serious challenge facing them is continuing their education while dealing with pregnancy and childrearing.

Teen Pregnancy And The Dropout Rate

About one-third of teenage girls who drop out of high school give pregnancy or parenthood as a major reason, according to the National Campaign to Prevent Teen and Unplanned Pregnancy. Just 40 percent of teenage mothers finish high school, only 34 percent earn either a high-school diploma or a General Educational Development (GED), and less than 2 percent of those who have a baby before the age of 18 finish college by age 30.

This leaves teen mothers at a tremendous economic and social disadvantage in later life, making it more difficult for them to achieve personal and career goals and economic independence. But their children are also affected. The CDC notes that children of teenage mothers are less likely to succeed in school, are more likely to drop out of high school, have more health problems, are more likely to give birth as a teenager themselves and face unemployment as young adults. In order to break this cycle, it's critical for pregnant teens and teenage mothers to complete at least their high-school education and, ideally, go on to college or specialized job training.

Some communities offer dropout prevention programs for pregnant and parenting teens. These generally include multiple services, including remedial education classes, tutoring, vocational training, counseling, healthcare, child care, and transportation assistance. These programs typically last about a year and often take place at more than one community location.

The Education Rights Of Pregnant Or Parenting Teens

Pregnant teens and teenage mothers have the same rights as any other student to continue their education. Title IX of the Education Amendments of 1972 is a piece of legislation that prohibits discrimination and ensures the following rights:

- Pregnant or parenting students cannot be excluded from any educational program, including extracurricular activities like clubs, honor societies, homecoming activities, and sports.

- A school must make reasonable adjustments to accommodate a student's pregnancy status. For instance, a school may need to provide a larger than standard desk, allow frequent bathroom trips, or permit temporary access to an elevator, if available.

- Schools may implement special classes for pregnant students, but participation must be voluntary, and the educational curricula and programs must be comparable to those offered to other students.

- Any special services or considerations provided to other students with temporary medical conditions must also be provided to pregnant students. And a student who is pregnant must not be required to submit a doctor's note to participate in educational activities unless a note is also required of other students with conditions that require a doctor's care.

- A school must excuse a student's absence because of pregnancy or childbirth for as long as the student's doctor deems medically necessary. And when the student returns to school, she must be allowed to return to the same academic level as before her leave.

If you are a pregnant teen, and you believe your rights to an education under Title IX have been denied, you can file a complaint with the U.S. Department of Education's (ED) Office of Civil Rights (OCR) at the office's website, www.ed.gov/ocr/complaintintro.html. You can also lodge a complaint with your state's OCR office.

Education Options

Title IX specifies the rights of pregnant and parenting teens to continue their education at their local public school, but depending on where they live, there are likely other options and strategies to help these students meet challenges and ultimately complete their education. Examples include:

- **Specialized schools.** Although the days of shipping pregnant teens off to isolated schools are long gone, in some cases it may be possible to choose a different school that's better equipped with services like prenatal care, parenting classes, knowledgeable staff and counselors, and day-care centers.

- **Online education or distance learning.** There are a number of fully accredited options for online or distance education that are available to pregnant or parenting teens. Some offer general academic curricula, while some are dedicated to special programs, but they generally work through websites, email correspondence, and/or webinars.

- **Homeschooling.** It's not for everyone, but some pregnant and parenting teens and their own parents have found that homeschooling can work well for all or part of their remaining education. Homeschools are regulated by the individual states, so requirements and policies vary, but they do have the advantage of increased schedule flexibility.

- **Residential treatment center.** In cases where a pregnant teen is also experiencing serious medical or emotional issues, many residential facilities offer programs that allow students to continue their education while receiving the treatment they need.

- **Switch from private to public school.** Private schools that don't receive federal funding are not necessarily bound by the provisions of Title IX. If a pregnant or parenting teen is enrolled in such a school, a move to a local public school can help ensure that she has access to the necessary accommodations for a quality education.

- **Support groups.** Many states, communities, and local organizations offer different types of support groups for pregnant and parenting teens. Depression, anxiety, and other emotional issues often go along with these situations, and discussing challenges with counselors and with others in similar circumstances can help lessen fears and provide valuable insight into managing these issues while continuing their education.

References

1. "Continuing Education For Teen Parents," Pregnancybirthbaby.org.au, June 2015.

2. "Drop Out Rates Among Pregnant Teens," Teenpregnancystatistics.org, 2009.

3. "Finishing School As A Mom," Teenpregnancystatistics.org, 2009.

4. Malone, Gloria. "High Schools Need To Support Teen Mothers," America.aljazeera.com, June 20, 2015.

5. "Pregnant? A Teen Parent? Protect Your Future: Stay In School," Publiccounsel.org, Fall, 2016.

6. Shuger, Lisa. "Teen Pregnancy And High School Dropout: What Communities Can Do To Address These Issues," National Campaign to Prevent Teen and Unplanned Pregnancy, 2012.

7. "Supporting The Academic Success Of Pregnant And Parenting Students," U.S. Department of Education (ED), June 2013.

8. "Teen Pregnancy Statistics," Teenhelp.com, 2016.

9. Van Pelt, Jennifer, MA. "Keeping Teen Moms In School: A School Social Work Challenge," Socialworktoday.com, March/April 2012.

Chapter 58

Considering Emancipation From Your Parents

Facing a pregnancy forces teenagers to grow up quickly, take on new responsibilities, and make adult decisions. Ideally, you will receive support and guidance from your parents during this challenging time. In some cases, however, teen pregnancy can create a rift within a family, especially when you and your parents disagree about the best course of action to take. If the situation at home becomes impossible to handle, one possible option for teenagers to consider is emancipation.

Emancipation is a legal procedure that allows someone under the age of 18 to be officially released from their parents' custody and control. Although you are still a minor, emancipation means that you assume legal authority for yourself and gain the right to make decisions without the consent or approval of your parents. This includes decisions relating to pregnancy, such as whether to have an abortion, continue a pregnancy, or place a baby for adoption. Once emancipated, however, you must also take full responsibility for your own food, clothing, housing, transportation, education, and medical care. Your parents are no longer required to provide you with a place to live or financial support.

> ## Did You Know...
> Emancipation does not grant a teenager all of the privileges of adulthood. No matter their legal status, minors cannot drive a car until age 16, vote or buy tobacco products until age 18, and drink alcohol until age 21.

"Considering Emancipation From Your Parents," © 2017 Omnigraphics. Reviewed March 2017.

Getting pregnant and having a baby does not automatically make you emancipated. Instead, you have to petition a court, present evidence of your maturity and ability to support yourself, and receive a declaration of emancipation from a judge. The only ways for a teenager to be emancipated without a judicial order are to get married or join the military. Although being pregnant does not change your legal status, some states have laws granting minors the right to control decisions about their own pregnancy, including making independent choices about abortion and adoption.

Reasons For Emancipation

Many teenagers have trouble getting along with their parents, and the tension and conflict can create a strong desire to leave home and live independently. If you believe you would be better off living apart from your parents, you have a number of options. You could start by talking to a school social worker about family counseling services that might help you and your parents communicate better. Or your parents might agree to a formal or informal arrangement where you live temporarily with a responsible friend or relative who is willing to take care of you. If your situation at home is so bad that you feel unsafe, you can contact your state's department of social services or child protective services. If they determine that your family environment is unsuitable, they can find you alternative living arrangements, such as foster care or a group home.

Since gaining legal emancipation can be an expensive and complicated process, it may not be the best option for everyone. But there are a number of reasons you may want to consider seeking emancipation from your parents, including the following:

- they have threatened or abused you;

- they have denied you food or otherwise neglected you;

- they have kicked you out of the house;

- they have pressured or forced you to participate in illegal activities;

- they have lied to you or stolen from you;

- your home is unsanitary or unsafe.

The Emancipation Process

To gain legal emancipation before the age of 18, you have to file a petition in a family court. The minimum age to petition for emancipation varies by state, but in most cases you must be at least 16. The petition can be filed by you or by your parents, if they have accepted your decision to live separately. Since the forms can be confusing, it may be helpful to hire a family law attorney. In some states, teenagers who are seeking emancipation are eligible for free legal aid.

After submitting the paperwork, the next step is to collect documentation to prove that you meet the conditions for emancipation. You will need evidence that you have a place to live, such as an apartment lease, as well as proof that you can support yourself financially, such as an employment contract and bank statements. Basically, the judge will want to see that you are capable of living on your own as an adult.

Finally, you will need to appear before the judge in a court hearing. If your parents refuse to consent to the emancipation proceedings, you will have to convince the judge that denying your petition would cause you significant harm. If the judge grants your request for emancipation, you will receive an official decree from the court indicating your legal status as an independent adult. You can show a copy of the decree to anyone who requests parental permission, such as schools, employers, landlords, or doctors.

Rights And Responsibilities

Emancipation and legal adulthood give you new rights, as well as new responsibilities. You can sign a lease and get your own apartment, for instance, but you are also responsible for paying the rent and utility bills. You can also make your own decisions as far as your medical treatment, such as prenatal care, but you are also responsible for carrying health insurance and paying medical bills. You can also obtain a driver's license and enroll in college without approval from your parents.

It is important to note that emancipation only lasts as long as you continue to live independently as an adult. If you accept financial support from your parents or move back home, your legal status will revert to a dependent minor.

References

1. Alexander, Gemma. "How to Help a Teen Get Emancipated," Avvo, October 21, 2016.

2. LaMance, Ken. "Emancipation Lawyers," LegalMatch, 2017.

3. "The Post-Divorce-Parenting Glossary: Emancipation," Custody Zen, 2017.

Chapter 59
Finding A Place To Live

For pregnant teenagers and young parents, finding a place to live can sometimes be difficult. Although studies suggest that living at home with your parents is often the best option, you may be unable to do so for reasons of financial hardship, overcrowding, or abuse or neglect. Some of the alternative living arrangements that may be available include a friend or relative's home, a maternity group home, foster care, or a rental unit.

Living With Your Parents

If you are under the age of 18 and unmarried, you are considered a dependent minor. This legal status means that your parents are required by law to meet your basic needs for food, shelter, and supervision. Their responsibility to take care of you does not end when you become pregnant or give birth to a baby. It is against the law for your parents to kick you out of the house without making arrangements for another safe place for you to live.

Many experts believe that pregnant and parenting teens should keep living at home if possible. Studies have shown that young mothers who continue to live at home with their parents are more likely to finish high school, which gives them more opportunities for success in the future. As a result, many laws and government-funded assistance programs are designed to encourage young mothers to live at home. For instance, the federal Temporary Assistance to Needy Families (TANF) program requires unmarried parents under age 17 to live with a parent or guardian and to be enrolled in school to qualify for benefits.

In some cases, however, living at home may not be an acceptable option—especially if you and your parents disagree about how to handle your pregnancy. Although your parents have a duty to provide shelter and supervision until you turn 18, the law does not require them

"Finding A Place To Live," © 2017 Omnigraphics. Reviewed March 2017.

to let you live in their home. Your parents may decide to make arrangements for you to stay somewhere else that will meet your basic needs, such as a friend or relative's house, a maternity group home, or a boarding school. As long as you are a dependent minor, you are expected to live where your parents say you should live.

Your parents' rights and responsibilities are much more limited when it comes to your child (their grandchild). Even if you live at home, your parents are not legally required to provide shelter or financial support for your baby. If your parents decide that you should live elsewhere, they are only allowed to keep your child at home with them under certain conditions:

- if you give them permission to do so;

- if a family court or the department of social services has awarded them custody; or

- if you are unable to care for the child because you are in a hospital, treatment facility, juvenile detention facility, jail, or prison.

Exploring Other Options

If you must move out of your parents' home, it is important to come up with a plan. Otherwise you may end up "couch surfing," or staying with a series of friends and relatives on a short-term basis. Moving around can make it difficult for you to stay in school, keep a job, get to doctor appointments, and be eligible for benefits such as TANF and Medicaid. It may be helpful to work with a trustworthy adult to find somewhere safe to stay where all your needs will be met. Experts suggest talking to a school counselor, a social worker at the local health department, or a youth outreach person at a recreation center or church.

If you decided to leave your parents' home because you felt unsafe—or you felt that your child's physical or emotional health was at risk—you should contact the police or the state department of social services. If a state agency investigates the situation and determines that it is not in your best interest to live with your parents, the state must help you find a suitable, adult-supervised living arrangement.

Many local governments and nonprofit organizations offer programs to help pregnant and parenting youth who lack appropriate housing or are homeless. Some of these programs go beyond simply providing shelter and offer a variety of resources and support services to help you take care of yourself and your baby. Some of the supportive housing options available include:

- **Maternity Group Homes**

   Also known as Second Chance Homes, these facilities provide adult-supervised housing for young parents and their children who are unable to live at home due to abuse or neglect. They offer residents access to such services as counseling, education, job training, employment assistance, daycare, healthcare, and transportation.

- **Transitional Housing**

  These programs have been established by many state governments to provide shelter and support to adolescent parents. Some facilities offer meals and shelter on a short-term, emergency basis, while others offer additional services to help teens learn to live independently, such as educational assessment and referrals, career training and job placement, and rental assistance.

- **Foster Care**

  Some teens enter the foster care system when they become pregnant, while others become pregnant when they are already in foster care. Most state systems place a strong emphasis on keeping young mothers together with their children to promote healthy bonding and attachment. They offer placements and support services to help young parents learn to care for their babies and become successful parents, ranging from specially trained foster home environments to residential treatment facilities.

Did You Know...

According to the U.S. Department of Health and Human Services (HHS), 80 percent of teenage mothers who are homeless cannot find stable, long-term living arrangements. Yet many homeless shelters and battered women's shelters do not accept teenage mothers or their young children.

Renting A Place

Renting an apartment, house, or mobile home is an attractive option for young parents who are eager to live independently as a family unit. Since minors under the age of 18 are not legally responsible for contracts they sign, however, most property owners, rental agents, and utility companies will not sign agreements with a minor. In addition, minors are not eligible for public assistance for housing because the federal government prefers that they live at home with a parent or guardian.

Your main option for renting a place of your own is to have an adult friend or relative sign a lease on your behalf. A lease is a legal contract between the owner of the property (landlord) and the person renting the property (tenant) that establishes the rights and responsibilities of each party. It should describe the property, list the amount of the rent and how often it must be paid, and indicate the term or length of the agreement. It should also say whether a security deposit is required and explain who is responsible for arranging and paying for utilities, such as water, heat, and electricity. It is important to understand that the adult who signs the lease assumes full legal responsibility for paying the rent and for any damage to the property. You and your child are listed as occupants.

References

1. Desiderio, Gina. "Helping Pregnant and Parenting Teens Find Housing," Healthy Teen Network, October 7, 2014.

2. "Pregnancy and Parenting: A Legal Guide for Adolescents," University of North Carolina, 2006.

Chapter 60

Second Chance Homes

Second Chance Homes are adult-supervised, supportive group homes or apartment clusters for teen mothers and their children who cannot live at home because of abuse, neglect or other extenuating circumstances. Second Chance Homes can also offer supports to help young families become self-sufficient and reduce the risk of repeat pregnancies. They provide a home where teen mothers can live, but they also offer program services to help put young mothers and their children on the path to a better future. Several federal resources are available to help state and local governments and community-based organizations create Second Chance Homes that provide safe, stable, nurturing environments for teen mothers and their children.

Second Chance Homes programs vary across the country, but generally include:

- An adult-supervised, supportive living arrangement

- Pregnancy prevention services or referrals

- A requirement to finish high school or obtain a General Educational Development (GED)

- Access to support services such as child care, healthcare, transportation, and counseling

- Parenting and life skills classes

- Education, job training, and employment services

- Community involvement

- Individual case management and mentoring

About This Chapter: This chapter includes text excerpted from "About Second Chance Homes," U.S. Department of Housing and Urban Development (HUD), October 16, 2016.

- Culturally sensitive services

- Services to ensure a smooth transition to independent living

Why Are They Important?

Second Chance Homes offer a nurturing home for society's most vulnerable families, teen mothers and their children with nowhere else to go. Almost half of all poor children under six are born to adolescent parents. Children of teen mothers are 50 percent more likely to have low birthweight, 33 percent more likely to become teen mothers themselves, and 2.7 times more likely to be incarcerated than the sons of mothers who delay childbearing. Teen mothers are half as likely to earn their high school diplomas or GEDs and are more likely to be on welfare than mothers who are older when they give birth. In addition, research shows that over 60 percent of teen parents have experienced sexual and/or physical abuse, often by a household member. Limited early findings indicate that residents of Second Chance Homes have fewer repeat pregnancies, better high school/GED completion rates, stronger life skills, increased self-sufficiency, and healthier babies.

Second Chance Homes help teen mothers and their children comply with welfare reform requirements. Under the 1996 welfare law, an unmarried parent under 18 cannot receive welfare assistance unless she lives with a parent, guardian or adult relative. However, if such a living arrangement is inappropriate (for example, if her family's whereabouts are unknown or if she was abused), states may waive the rule and either determine her current living arrangement to be appropriate, or help her find an alternative adult-supervised supportive living arrangement such as a Second Chance Home. Also, in states where alternatives such as Second Chance Homes are currently not available, teen mothers could be forced to choose between inappropriate living arrangements and losing their cash assistance. Making Second Chance Homes available to teen mothers in need could provide these teens with stable housing, case management, and preparation for independent living.

Second Chance Homes can support teen families who are homeless or in foster care. State foster care systems may not have the capacity to place the teens and their children together, and frequently, homeless shelters, battered women's shelters, and transitional living facilities cannot accept teen parents under age 17. Unfortunately, homelessness poses the threat of separation in young families. For vulnerable families with no safe, stable places to go, Second Chance Homes can help fill the gap.

Who Is Eligible?

Eligibility criteria for Second Chance Homes vary from program to program. Some programs are targeted for adolescent mothers (between the ages of 14 to 20, for example), mothers receiving welfare assistance, or homeless families. Other programs are open to any mother in need of a place to live—regardless of age, income or the assistance program for which she qualifies. Teen mothers can be referred to Second Chance Homes through welfare agencies, homeless shelters, or foster care programs, or by community organizations, schools, clinics, or hospitals. Mothers may also self-refer.

Where Are They?

Nationwide, at least 6 states have made a statewide commitment to Second Chance Home programs: Massachusetts, Nevada, New Mexico, Rhode Island, Texas, and Georgia. In statewide networks, community-based organizations operate the homes under contract to the states and deliver the services. States share in the cost of the program, refer teens to homes, and set standards and guidelines for services to teen families. In addition, there are many local Second Chance Home programs operating in an estimated 25 additional states.

Chapter 61

Health Insurance During Pregnancy

Health insurance helps you pay for medical services and sometimes prescription drugs. Once you purchase insurance coverage, you and your health insurer each agree to pay a part of your medical expenses—usually a certain dollar amount or percentage of the expenses.

How To Get Health Coverage

You can get healthcare coverage through:

- A group coverage plan at your job or your spouse or partner's job

- Your parents' insurance plan, if you are under 26 years old

- A plan you purchase on your own directly from a health insurance company or through the Health Insurance Marketplace

- Government programs such as Medicare, Medicaid, or Children's Health Insurance Program (CHIP)

- The Veterans Administration or TRICARE for military personnel

- Your state, if it provides a health insurance plan

- Continuing employer coverage from your former employer, on a temporary basis under the Consolidated Omnibus Budget Reconciliation Act (COBRA)

About This Chapter: Text in this chapter begins with excerpts from "Finding Health Insurance," USA.gov, December 19, 2016; Text beginning with the heading "Private Health Plans And Pregnancy" is excerpted from "Health Coverage If You're Pregnant Or Plan To Get Pregnant," Centers for Medicare and Medicaid Services (CMS), March 16, 2017.

Types Of Health Insurance Plans

When purchasing health insurance, your choices typically fall into one of three categories:

- Traditional fee-for-service health insurance plans are usually the most expensive choice, but they offer you the most flexibility in choosing healthcare providers.

- Health maintenance organizations (HMOs) offer lower co-payments and cover the costs of more preventive care, but your choice of healthcare providers is limited to those who are part of the plan.

- Preferred provider organizations (PPOs) offer lower co-payments like HMOs but give you more flexibility in selecting a provider.

Choosing A Health Insurance Plan

Read the fine print when choosing among different healthcare plans. Also ask a lot of questions, such as:

- Do I have the right to go to any doctor, hospital, clinic, or pharmacy I choose?

- Are specialists, such as eye doctors and dentists, covered?

- Does the plan cover special conditions or treatments such as pregnancy, psychiatric care, and physical therapy?

- Does the plan cover home care or nursing home care?

- Will the plan cover all medications my physician may prescribe?

- What are the deductibles? Are there any co-payments? Deductibles are the amount you must pay before your insurance company will pay a claim. These differ from co-payments, which are the amount of money you pay when you receive medical services or a prescription.

- What is the most I will have to pay out of my own pocket to cover expenses?

- If there is a dispute about a bill or service, how is it handled?

Health Coverage If You're Pregnant Or Plan To Get Pregnant

All Health Insurance Marketplace and Medicaid plans cover pregnancy and childbirth. This is true even if your pregnancy begins before your coverage takes effect.

> **Important:** Having a baby qualifies you for a Special Enrollment Period (SEP).
>
> This means that after you have your baby you can enroll in or change Marketplace coverage even if it's outside the Open Enrollment Period. When you enroll in the new plan, your coverage can be effective from the day the baby was born.

If you already have Marketplace coverage when your baby is born, you can do one of 2 things:

- Keep your current plan and add your child to your coverage.

- Change to a different Marketplace plan.

Private Health Plans And Pregnancy

- Maternity care and childbirth—services provided before and after your child is born—are essential health benefits. This means all qualified health plans inside and outside the Marketplace must cover them.

- You get this coverage even if you were pregnant before your coverage starts. Under the healthcare law pre-existing conditions are covered, including pregnancy.

- Health plans sold inside and outside the Marketplace must provide a Summary of Benefits and Coverage document. Page 7 of most summaries spells out how plans cover the costs of childbirth.

- Some grandfathered individual health plans—the kind you buy yourself, not the kind you get through a job—aren't required to cover pregnancy and childbirth. If you have a grandfathered individual plan, contact your insurance company to learn about your pregnancy and childbirth coverage.

Maternity And Childbirth Under Medicaid And CHIP

Maternity care and childbirth are covered by Medicaid and Children's Health Insurance Program (CHIP).

These state-based programs cover pregnant women and their children below certain income levels. Eligibility and benefits are different in each state. Income levels to qualify are different for Medicaid and CHIP.

Having a baby
(normal delivery)

- Amount owed to providers: $7,540
- Plan pays $5,490
- Patient pays $2,050

Sample care costs:

Hospital charges (mother)	$2,700
Routine obstetric care	$2,100
Hospital charges (baby)	$900
Anesthesia	$900
Laboratory tests	$500
Prescriptions	$200
Radiology	$200
Vaccines, other preventive	$40
Total	**$7,540**

Patient pays:

Deductibles	$700
Copays	$30
Coinsurance	$1320
Limits or exclusions	$0
Total	**$2,050**

Figure 61.1. Summary Of Benefits And Coverage: What This Health Plan Covers And What It Costs

This example shows how this plan might cover medical care in given situations. Use this example to see, in general, how much financial protection a patient might get if they are covered under different plans.

NOTE: This Is Not A Cost Estimator. Don't use this example to estimate your actual costs under this plan. The actual care you receive will be different from this example, and the cost of that care will also be different.

(Source: "Insurance Company 1: Plan Option 1," Centers for Medicare and Medicaid Services (CMS).)

You can apply for Medicaid or CHIP any time during the year, not just during Marketplace Open Enrollment. You can apply 2 ways: Directly through your state agency, or by filling out a Marketplace application.

More People Qualify For Medicaid

Many states have expanded their Medicaid programs to cover all people whose income is below certain levels. Even if you didn't qualify for coverage in the past, you may qualify now.

Whether you qualify for Medicaid depends on whether your state has expanded Medicaid coverage and your household size and income.

Chapter 62

WIC: The Special Supplemental Nutrition Program For Women, Infants, And Children

What Is Women, Infants, And Children (WIC)?

Women, Infants, And Children (WIC) was established as a permanent program in 1974 to safeguard the health of low-income women, infants, and children up to age 5 who are at nutritional risk. This mission is carried out by providing nutritious foods to supplement diets, nutrition education (including breastfeeding promotion and support), and referrals to health and other social services.

Where Is WIC Available?

The program is available in all 50 States, 34 Indian Tribal Organizations (ITO), American Samoa (AS), District of Columbia (DC), Guam (GU), Commonwealth of the Northern Mariana Islands (CNMI), Puerto Rico (PR), and the Virgin Islands (VI). While funded through grants from the Federal Government, WIC is administered by 90 State agencies, with services provided at a variety of clinic locations including, but not limited to, county health departments, hospitals, schools, and Indian Health Service (IHS) facilities.

What Food Benefits Do WIC Participants Receive?

The foods provided through the WIC Program are designed to supplement participants' diets with specific nutrients. WIC authorized foods include infant cereal, baby foods,

About This Chapter: This chapter includes text excerpted from "The Special Supplemental Nutrition Program For Women, Infants And Children (WIC Program)," Food and Nutrition Service (FNS), U.S. Department of Agriculture (USDA), February 6, 2015.

iron-fortified adult cereal, fruits and vegetables, vitamin C-rich fruit or vegetable juice, eggs, milk, cheese, yogurt, soy-based beverages, tofu, peanut butter, dried and canned beans/peas, canned fish, whole wheat bread and other whole-grain options. For infants of women who do not fully breastfeed, WIC provides iron-fortified infant formula. Special infant formulas and medical foods may also be provided if medically indicated.

Program benefits include more than food.

WIC benefits are not limited only to food. Participants have access to a number of resources, including health screening, nutrition and breastfeeding counseling, immunization screening and referral, substance abuse referral, and more.

Am I Eligible?

Pregnant, postpartum, and breastfeeding women, infants, and children up to age 5 who meet certain requirements are eligible. These requirements include income eligibility and State residency. Additionally, the applicant must be individually determined to be at "nutrition risk" by a health professional or a trained health official.

How WIC Helps

WIC supplemental foods have shown to provide wide ranging benefits. They include longer, safer pregnancies, with fewer premature births and infant deaths; improved dietary outcomes for infants and children; improved maternal health; and improved performance at school, among others. In addition to health benefits, WIC participants showed significant savings in healthcare costs when compared to non-participants.

What Is "Nutrition Risk" And Why Is It Important?

Two major types of nutrition risk are recognized for WIC eligibility: medically-based risks such as anemia, underweight, history of pregnancy complications, or poor pregnancy outcomes; and dietary risks, such as inappropriate nutrition/feeding practices or failure to meet the current Dietary Guidelines for Americans (DGA). Women, infants, and children at nutrition risk have much greater risk of experiencing health problems.

I'm Eligible, What Do I Do Next?

Those who are interested in applying for benefits should contact their State agency to request information on where to schedule an appointment. Applicants will be advised on what to bring to the appointment in order to verify eligibility.

EBT makes it easier to use food benefits.

In most WIC State agencies, participants receive paper checks or vouchers to purchase food, while a few distribute food through centralized warehouses or deliver the foods to participants' homes. However, all WIC State agencies have been mandated to implement WIC electronic benefit transfer (EBT) statewide by October 1, 2020. EBT uses a magnetic stripe or smart card, similar to a credit card, that participants use in the check-out lane to redeem their food benefits. EBT provides a safer, easier, and more efficient grocery experience and provides greater flexibility in the way WIC participants can shop.

Focus on breastfeeding.

Even though breast milk is the most nutritious and complete source of food for infants, nationally less than 30 percent of infants are breastfed at 1 year of age. A major goal of the WIC Program is to improve the nutritional status of infants; therefore, WIC mothers are encouraged to breastfeed their infants, unless medically contraindicated. Pregnant women and new WIC mothers are provided breastfeeding educational materials and support through counseling and guidance.

WIC Facts

- If you participate in another assistance program you may be automatically income-eligible for WIC.

- Breastfeeding mothers are eligible to participate in WIC longer than non-breastfeeding mothers.

- More than half of the infants in the United States participate in WIC.

- WIC participants support the local economy through their purchases.

- WIC works with farmers markets to help increase participant access to provide fresh, locally grown fruits and vegetables.

Chapter 63

Vaccines For Uninsured Children

The Vaccines for Children (VFC) Program provides vaccines to children whose parents or guardians may not be able to afford them. This helps ensure that all children have a better chance of getting their recommended vaccinations on schedule. These vaccines protect babies, young children, and adolescents from 16 diseases.

Who Is Eligible For The VFC Program?

Any child that is younger than 19 years of age and meets one of the following requirements:

- Medicaid-eligible

- Uninsured

- American Indian or Alaska Native

- Underinsured*

Underinsured children are eligible to receive vaccines only at Federally Qualified Health Centers (FQHC) or Rural Health Clinics (RHC). FQHCs and RHCs provide healthcare to medically under-served areas and meet certain criteria under Medicare and Medicaid programs.

What Is "Underinsured"?

Underinsured means your child has health insurance, but it:

- doesn't cover vaccines, or

- doesn't cover certain vaccines.

About This Chapter: This chapter includes text excerpted from "VFC Program," Centers for Disease Control and Prevention (CDC), February 16, 2016.

What Is The Cost?

There is no charge for the vaccines given by a VFC provider to eligible children. But there can be some other costs with the visit:

- Doctors can charge a set (or standard) fee to administer each shot.

- There can be a fee for the office visit.

- There can be fees for non-vaccine services, like an eye exam or blood test.

Where Can My Child Get Vaccinated?

Nationally, there are nearly 44,000 healthcare providers enrolled in the VFC Program. If your child is VFC-eligible, ask your child's doctor if they are a VFC provider. For help finding a VFC provider near you, contact your state or local health department's VFC Program Coordinator, or call Centers for Disease Control and Prevention (CDC) at 800-CDC-INFO (800-232-4636) for assistance.

Federal Funding, State Management

The VFC Program is funded through the Centers for Medicare and Medicaid Services (CMS) to the Centers for Disease Control and Prevention (CDC). In general, state health departments manage the VFC Program, but in some locations it may be managed by a city or territorial health department.

Diseases that are preventable by recommended childhood vaccines recommended by the Advisory Committee on Immunization Practices (ACIP) include the following.

- Diphtheria
- Haemophilus influenzae type b (Hib)
- Hepatitis A
- Hepatitis B
- Human Papillomavirus (HPV)
- Influenza (flu)
- Measles
- Meningococcal

- Mumps
- Pertussis (whooping cough)
- Pneumococcal
- Polio
- Rotavirus
- Rubella (German Measles)
- Tetanus (lockjaw)
- Varicella (chickenpox)

(Source: "VFC Detailed Questions And Answers For Parents," Centers for Disease Control and Prevention (CDC).)

Chapter 64

Understanding Child Care Options

Looking for child care for the first time can be an unfamiliar experience that raises many questions. Questions that leave you wondering, "Will I be able to find care for my child(ren)? Where do I start?"

Together with local Child Care Resource & Referral agencies, Child Care Aware® helps parents become informed consumers of child care. One way we do this is by answering your child care questions.

What Types Of Child Care Are There?

Not all child care programs are the same. Different families have different needs. Below you will find various descriptions of child care programs. Your local Child Care Resource & Referral (CCR&R) will work with you to determine what programs are available in your area.

- **Child Care Center:** A nonresidential program, often with children separated by classrooms or age groups. Child care centers have program directors, lead teachers and assistant teachers, and additional staff. Child care centers are likely to offer children a structured curriculum.

- **Family Child Care Home:** Child care offered in a provider's home. You see more mixed ages in a Family Child Care setting. Staff includes the provider/owner and maybe one or two additional staff. Family Child Care providers may or may not offer a structured curriculum.

About This Chapter: Text in this chapter is excerpted from "Putting The Pieces Together Solving The Child Care Puzzle," © 2010-2017 National Association of Child Care Resource & Referral Agencies (NACCRRA). Reprinted with permission.

- **Preschool/PreK*/Prekindergarten:** An early education program for children ages 3–5. Preschool programs offer curriculum to help your child prepare for school. Some child care programs may refer to the 3–5 year old classroom as the PreK classroom.

  - **Part-Day Preschool:** A program 2–3 hours a day, for 3–5 days a week. These programs focus on early education and school readiness. With a part-day preschool program, you may need to look for additional child care options to accommodate your work schedule and the schedule of the program. These programs may be available to all families.

  - **State-Funded Prekindergarten Programs:** Programs targeting children ages 3–5, focusing on early education and school readiness. Some states offer these programs at either a low or no cost to eligible families. Programs may be part day or a full school day. With a state-funded prekindergarten program, you may need to look for additional child care options to accommodate your work schedule and the schedule of the program.

* It is always important to clarify what a particular program means when someone refers to "PreK."

- **Head Start Programs:** Child development programs funded by the U.S. Department of Health and Human Services (HHS). These comprehensive programs offer an educational setting, health and nutrition information, and various parent involvement opportunities. Head Start programs typically have income eligibility guidelines.

- **Inclusive Child Care:** Programs that offer child care services to families of children with special needs. These programs strive to keep all children in a common environment or classroom. Inclusive programs eliminate the separation of typically developing children and children with special needs.

What Age Group Is Your Child In?

In different child care settings, the age of your child may determine what classroom or group he is in. It may also affect the amount you pay for child care. It is good to familiarize yourself with these age classifications.

- **Infants:** Birth to age 12–18 months (may vary by setting)

- **Toddlers:** 12–18 months to 36 months

- **Preschoolers:** 3 to 5 years old

- **School-age:** 5 to 12 years old

What Help Is Available To Pay For Child Care?

At times, you may find yourself looking for help with your child care payments. Financial assistance options vary by location, but here are some examples that may be available to you.

- **State Programs:** Federally funded financial assistance programs, or subsidy programs, that pay a portion of an eligible family's child care fees. These programs are offered by state agencies and distributed through state or local programs. Income eligibility requirements vary by state.

- **Local Programs:** In some areas, there may be local programs available to your family that will assist with your child care costs. Programs may be offered through local governments, nonprofit agencies or service organizations.

- **Employer Programs:** Some employers may offer child care assistance through Dependent Care assistance accounts or other Employee Assistance Programs.

- **Provider Specific Programs:** Child care programs may offer financial assistance for families. Incentives to ask a prospective provider about include sliding fee scales, scholarships or sibling discounts.

- **Tax Credits:** There are various tax credits your family might be eligible for if you have qualifying children.
  - Earned Income Tax Credit
  - Child Tax Credit
  - Child and Dependent Care Tax Credit
  - State Tax Credits

Why Is Screening Important?

When you return to work or school, you want to know that you have selected the most suitable child care environment for your child. By screening prospective child care programs, you will have done your homework and made an informed child care choice.

- **Interview:** Visit with prospective child care providers and/or center directors and teachers. Get to know a little bit more about who will be caring for your child.

- **On-Site Visit:** Be sure to visit the child care program. You may visit more than once. You might want to visit one on one with the provider. You will also want to visit with children present. You will be able to observe caregiver and child interactions.

- **Training:** Learn about the training prospective providers have gone through to become a caregiver. Also ask about ongoing training opportunities.

- **Background Checks:** Check with both child care centers and family child care providers regarding the completion of background check on all individuals/staff that will have contact with your child.

- **References:** Speak to other families, both past and current, about their experiences in the program.

Who Regulates Child Care?

Regulations for child care vary from state to state. Each state has a regulatory agency that oversees the implementation and compliance of standards and guidelines set for local child care providers. In addition, child care providers and centers can voluntarily go through programs focusing on the quality of care being offered to families.

- **Licensed:** States have regulations in place for licensing child care centers and family child care homes. It is important that you check to see what the regulations are in your state. Your local Child Care Resource and Referral agency will be able to assist you with this information.

- **Licensed-Exempt:** In some states, certain types of programs are not required to be licensed. These programs may include family child care homes with six or fewer children, religious–based child care programs and programs offered in public schools.

- **Accreditation:** A voluntary program requiring child care providers to meet specific nationally recognized performance standards. These standards generally exceed state licensing requirements. Some accrediting organizations include:

  - National Association for the Education of Young Children (NAEYC) (www.naeyc.org)

  - National Accreditation Commission for Early Care and Education Programs (NAC) (www.naccp.org)

  - National Early Childhood Program Accreditation (NECPA) (www.necpa.net)

  - National Association of Family Child Care (NAFCC) (www.nafcc.org)

  - Council on Accreditation (COA) www.coanet.org

- **Quality Rating and Improvement Systems (QRIS):** Statewide or local programs created to improve the quality and affordability of child care. The focus of these programs is consumer education benchmarks and tiered reimbursement programs. Now that you are prepared to begin your search for child care, keep in mind the choices you make will impact your child's future. Your child care provider will work with you as your child's nurturer, educator and cheerleader when you are not there to care for your child. Maintaining a solid, consistent, long-term relationship will positively impact your child's early experiences and preparation for school.

What Are You Looking For?

There are many terms associated with the full- or part-time care of your child. Most commonly, you might hear "child care" or "day care."

- **Child Care, Day Care, Early Care and Education programs:** Full-time care and supervision of your child(ren), typically between 6:00 a.m. and 6:00 p.m. These programs offer safe, structured learning environments that help prepare your child for school.

- **Babysitter:** Care offered on an as-needed basis through a friend, neighbor or young adult in your area. You may look for a babysitter when you need to run an errand in the evening or on the weekend.

When Do You Need Child Care?

Families' schedules vary. You know best when you will need child care to accommodate everyone's schedule.

- **Traditional Hours:** Traditional hours include the 8:00 a.m. to 5:00 p.m. work day, with time allotted for pick up and drop off. Generally, a child care program offering care during traditional hours might be open from 6:00 a.m. to 6:00 p.m.

- **Nontraditional Hours:** This type of care may be more appealing to shift workers and families needing child care in the evenings and on the weekends. Nontraditional hours may include overnight or after-hours care.

- **Irregular Duty:** Families needing care for irregular duty may need a child care provider who can accommodate their nontraditional work schedule. Examples of irregular duty may include a rotating schedule with four days on shift, four days off shift.

Chapter 65

Finding Help Paying For Child Care

Your Child Is Priceless . . .

But paying for good child care can be a struggle. In fact, child care is probably the second largest expense in your budget after rent or mortgage payments.

By following these steps to child care budgeting, you may be able to reduce child care costs or get some help paying child care bills.

Five Steps To Healthy Child Care Budgeting

1. Plan Ahead

Start thinking about child care options and cost as far in advance as you can. No matter what type of care you are considering—a child care center, care in someone's home, or care for an infant, toddler, preschooler or school age child—finding the right child care option or help with child care expenses can take some time.

2. Call the Experts

Begin the search by calling your local experts—your Child Care Resource & Referral agency (CCR&R). CCR&Rs can give you the facts about child care. They can also provide a list of child care options and available financial assistance in your area.

About This Chapter: Text in this chapter is excerpted from "Finding Help Paying For Child Care," © 2010-2017 National Association of Child Care Resource & Referral Agencies (NACCRRA). Reprinted with permission.

3. Be A Smart Consumer

When you are at work, you want to know that your child is getting the kind of high-quality care that all children need to be healthy, happy and ready for school.

The checklist below helps you evaluate the value of the child care you are buying for your family. You can use this checklist in a child care center, a family child care home (care in someone else's home), or for an in-home provider who comes to your home.

The money you pay goes toward the caregivers' salary and on-going education and training so they can meet your child's needs. Your child care fees also help purchase food, toys, equipment, supplies, and pays for insurance, rent or mortgage, and other necessary expenses.

Ask These Questions To Evaluate Your Child Care Options

- Does the person who will be caring for your child have special training in early childhood education, First Aid and CPR?
- How long has the child care provider been providing child care?
- If there is more than one child care provider in the setting, is the total number of children in the group still small (group size)?
- Is one child care provider caring for just a few children (low child/adult ratio)?
- If you are considering a more formal child care program, is it state licensed or regulated? Is it nationally accredited?
- Have satisfactory criminal history background checks been conducted on each adult present?
- Has the program been inspected by the licensing agency within the last 12 months?
- Does the child care provider welcome drop-in visits, parent ideas, and involvement?
- Does the child care provider get on the children's eye level to talk with them and give them lots of attention and encouragement?
- Are there planned activities for children to do as well as lots of time for free play?
- Are materials—such as books, blocks, toys and art supplies—available to children all day long?
- Does the place look clean and safe and does everyone wash his or her hands often?
- Does the child care provider have written policies and procedures, including emergency plans?
- Does the child care provider have references?
- You know your child best—will your child be happy there?

Once you have evaluated your options and decided on a child care setting, be an involved and informed consumer. Visit often and participate in events at your child's program. This sends a strong message to your child and your child's provider that you think what your child is doing and learning is important.

4. Find Out What Kind Of Help May Be Available

The following child care assistance programs help families with the high cost of child care. Each type of child care financial assistance has different qualifications, so work with your local CCR&R and your employer's human resources department to make sure you get all the facts.

State Child Care Subsidies

Child care subsidies are available in every state to help families with the cost of child care. Usually, child care subsidies are available for working families earning low incomes, receiving Temporary Assistance for Needy Families (TANF), or in some cases enrolled in school. If eligible, you will pay part of the cost while the rest is paid directly to your selected child care provider.

Employer/College Support

Your employer may provide child care scholarships, discounts to certain programs or on-site child care at reduced rates. Colleges or universities may also have programs to help with child care costs.

Child Care Program Assistance

Your child care provider may offer scholarships, discounts or a sliding fee scale.

Pre-Kindergarten (Pre-K) Programs

Many states offer free or low-cost prekindergarten programs for 3- and 4- year-old children. Eligibility requirements vary by state but the goal of all prekindergarten programs is to make sure that children are prepared for kindergarten. Public schools and other child care settings offer prekindergarten programs during school hours.

Head Start And Early Head Start

Head Start and Early Head Start are federally- and sometimes state-funded full- or part-day programs that provide free early education and other services to help meet the health and school readiness needs of children in income eligible families.

Federal Earned Income Tax Credit (EITC)

You may be able to lower your taxes and even get money back if you qualify for the EITC. To qualify, you must be working full- or part-time and make less than a certain amount based on family size. You do not have to owe any taxes to get a refund using EITC.

Federal Child Tax Credit (CTC)

If you have a dependent child under age 17, you may be eligible for the Child Tax Credit, which can be worth hundreds of dollars per child. The income eligibility for the CTC is much higher than for the Earned Income Tax Credit, but you still do not have to owe any taxes to use the Child Tax Credit.

Federal Child And Dependent Care Tax Credit

If you have a child under the age of 13, pay for child care and owe federal income taxes, you may be eligible for this tax credit.

State Earned Income And Dependent Care Tax Credits

Many states offer their own earned Income or Child and Dependent Care tax credits. These credits are similar to the federal ones. In some states, you do not have to owe any taxes to get the State Child and Dependent Care credit. You can get both federal and state Earned Income and Child and Dependent Care credits.

Dependent Care Assistance Programs (DCAPs)

Your employer may offer a Dependent Care Assistance Program, which allows you to have up to $5,000 a year deducted from your paycheck on a pre-tax basis. The money is placed in a special account to be used for child care tuition reimbursement. You should never put more money in this account than you will actually spend because you will lose unspent funds at the end of the year. You cannot claim any money you put in a DCAP for the Child and Dependent Care Tax Credit.

5. Consider All Options

Think about what your family needs and take a close look at your budget. Are there alternatives to paying full-time child care? Is it possible or desirable to work fewer hours? If you are in a two-parent household, can you work at different times and share some hours of child care? Could you share child care expenses with another family? The most important thing is that your family and child are healthy and happy. By planning, getting the facts and using all available resources—especially your local CCR&R—you are off to a good start in making the best choice for your family.

Chapter 66
Child Custody

Child custody is an arrangement determined by a family court that specifies who should have legal control and responsibility for a minor child under the age of 18. Child custody questions typically arise when a child's parents divorce, separate, end their relationship, die, or become incapable of caring for the child. Child custody can be a highly contentious and emotionally charged issue, but judges usually try to keep the best interests of the child in mind.

There are two main types of child custody: physical custody and legal custody. Physical custody refers to who the child lives with, while legal custody refers to who makes decisions about the child's upbringing. Both types of child custody can be further broken down into sole custody or joint custody. Sole custody means that one parent has the primary responsibility, while joint custody means that both parents share responsibility.

In many cases, a child's mother and father will have joint physical custody as well as joint legal custody. The child spends time with both parents, and they cooperate to make important decisions affecting the child's welfare. In other cases, one parent will have sole physical custody—meaning that the child lives primarily with that parent—while both parents share joint legal custody. In cases where one parent is absent or deemed unfit, the other parent will have sole physical and legal custody.

Did You Know...

According to the U.S. Census Bureau, there were 11 million single-parent households with children under 18 in the United States as of 2016. Of these households, 8.5 million were led by single mothers and 2.5 million by single fathers.

"Child Custody," © 2017 Omnigraphics. Reviewed March 2017.

Sole Physical Custody

Physical custody is the right to have your child live with you. If you have sole physical custody, you are known as the custodial parent. This means that you have the primary responsibility for meeting your child's basic needs—such as food, clothing, shelter, and safety—on a daily basis.

A judge will sometimes award sole physical custody when one parent is in a better position to care for the child. The court may decide that the other parent is unfit due to financial, drug, or alcohol problems. Other times, sole physical custody is awarded to one parent to give the child geographic stability. If the two parents live far apart, it may make sense for the child to live in a single location in order to attend school, form friendships, and be part of a community. If a child's parents are unmarried, the biological mother is usually awarded sole physical custody unless the biological father petitions a court for joint custody.

Visitation And Child Support

If you have sole physical custody, the child's other parent (known as the noncustodial parent) typically has visitation rights. The child lives with you permanently, but the child visits with the noncustodial parent for a limited amount of time on a regular schedule.

A typical visitation schedule might allow the noncustodial parent to see the child one night per week and every other weekend. The noncustodial parent might also be entitled to spend time with the child during the summer and on certain holidays. In cases where one parent is considered unfit or has never developed a relationship with the child, a judge may order supervised visitation. For the child's protection, the noncustodial parent spends time with the child in the presence of another adult or in a licensed facility.

Once the visitation schedule is approved by the court, both the custodial and noncustodial parent are legally required to follow it. You cannot refuse a scheduled visit with the noncustodial parent unless you believe it would endanger the child. Likewise, the noncustodial parent cannot take the child away from you without permission or keep the child longer than scheduled. Violating or interfering with visitation rights is a serious offense that can result in a contempt of court citation.

If one parent is awarded sole physical custody, the noncustodial parent is usually required to make child support payments to help cover the child's living expenses. The amount varies depending on state laws and the respective income of each parent. You can use child support payments for such expenses as food, clothing, education, daycare, and healthcare. Failure to pay court-ordered child support can result in such penalties as fines, withheld wages, suspension of a driver's license or passport, arrest, and imprisonment.

Joint Physical Custody

If you have joint physical custody, you and your child's other parent share responsibility for meeting your child's basic needs. Your child will live with you part-time, and with the other parent part-time, according to a regular schedule. Courts usually prefer to award joint physical custody because it enables both parents to maintain a relationship with the child. In addition, it divides the burden of raising the child between the two parents. Studies have shown that children tend to do better in joint custody arrangements except when there is a high level of conflict between the parents.

Joint physical custody arrangements work best when the two parents live relatively close to each other, especially once the child reaches school age. Otherwise, constantly shuttling back and forth between two homes can put a strain on the child. The child does not necessarily have to spend exactly 50 percent of the time with each parent in a joint custody arrangement. Some parents spend alternate days, weeks, or months with the child. One type of joint custody arrangement, known as a "bird's nest" arrangement, allows the child to remain in the family home while the parents take turns living there. Parents who share custody need to establish a schedule around the child's school hours and activities as well as their own work hours.

Legal Custody

Legal custody is the right to make decisions about various aspects of your child's upbringing, such as education, health, and welfare. If you are awarded sole legal custody of your child, you have the authority to decide what school your child attends, what religion your child practices, and what kind of medical care your child receives. You also have the right to decide how to discipline your child.

In most states, courts prefer to award joint legal custody, which gives both parents equal rights to make decisions about the child's upbringing. The general feeling is that it is better for both parents to be looking out for the child's welfare instead of just one. Many courts allow joint legal custody even when one parent has sole physical custody. Sole legal custody is typically only awarded when a court determines that one parent is unfit to make decisions on behalf of the child.

The Child Custody Agreement

Decisions regarding child custody can be made through informal agreements between the parents or through official rulings by a family court judge. Family courts try to determine the best interests of the child and forge a custody agreement that promotes the child's interests. Some of the factors used to decide on child custody arrangements include the following:

- the parent's relationship with the child;

- the parent's ability and willingness to provide for the child;

- the parent's ability to provide a stable living situation;

- the proximity of the parent's home to the child's school and activities;

- the level of cooperation or interference with the other parent's relationship with the child;

- the child's age;

- the child's preferences;

- any evidence of abuse or neglect.

Once the custody agreement is approved by a judge, it becomes a binding legal contract that both parents are required to follow. If you want to make changes later, you have to file a petition with the court. Experts recommend that you consult with a qualified family law attorney to ensure that your custody agreement promotes the best interests of you and your child.

References

1. Otterstrom, Kristina. "Child Custody and Child Visitation: Terms to Know," Lawyers.com, 2017.

2. Tsui, Edward. "Divorce and Child Custody: Everything You Need to Know," Expertise, May 14, 2015.

3. "The Various Types of Child Custody," FindLaw, 2017.

Chapter 67

Child Support

The child support program ensures noncustodial parents provide financial support for their children, primarily collected through payroll withholding. Child support payments lift approximately one million families out of poverty each year. Among poor single mothers with children that receive it, child support accounts for 41 percent of the family's income.

In 2015, the child support program collected $28.6 billion for almost 16 million children. Eighty-six percent of all child support cases had support orders in place, and nearly 72 percent of those cases had at least some payments during the year. The child support program collects $5.26 for every government dollar spent.

The final rule makes changes to increase the effectiveness of the child support program for all families, which will result in an increase in timely payments to families, a decline in the nonpayment rate, and an increase in the number of noncustodial parents working and supporting their children.

The new rule removes regulatory barriers to cost-effective approaches to give states needed flexibility to increase the accuracy and accountability of support orders. The changes are consistent with research evidence and knowledge in the field and informed by many successful state-led innovations over the past two decades.

The rule also increases program efficiency and simplifies operational requirements by removing outdated barriers to electronic communication and document management. Given

About This Chapter: Text in this chapter begins with excerpts from "Overview—Final Rule 2016 Flexibility, Efficiency, And Modernization In Child Support Enforcement Programs," Administration for Children and Families (ACF), U.S. Department of Health and Human Services (HHS), October 5, 2016; Text beginning with the heading "What Are The Steps To Collect Child Support?" is excerpted from "How To Get Child Support," Administration for Children and Families (ACF), U.S. Department of Health and Human Services (HHS), September 9, 2014.

that three-quarters of child support payments are collected by employers through payroll withholding, the rule standardizes and streamlines payment processing so employers are not unduly burdened. Most importantly, these new provisions and guidelines are expected to result in families receiving more consistent payment of child support.

The Flexibility, Efficiency, and Modernization in Child Support Programs Final Rule strengthens and updates the child support program by amending existing rules, some of which are 35 years old, to:

- Ensure child support obligations are accurate and based upon the noncustodial parents' ability to pay;
- Increase consistent, on time payments to families;
- Move nonpaying cases to paying status;
- Increase the number of noncustodial parents supporting their children;
- Improve child support collection rates;
- Reduce the accumulation of unpaid and uncollectible child support arrearages; and
- Incorporate technological advances and evidence-based standards that support good customer service and cost-effective management practices.

What Are The Steps To Collect Child Support?

Typically it begins by identifying the father, often called establishing paternity. Once we know who the father is, a child support order is established and the child support agency can begin collecting and enforcing the child support order.

1. **Establish Fatherhood**

   If you were not married when your child was born, the first step is to—legally determining the father of the child. Many men will voluntarily acknowledge paternity.

   If a man is not certain that he is the father, the child support agency can arrange for genetic testing. These tests are simple to take and highly accurate. Either parent can request a blood test in contested paternity cases.

2. **Establish A Child Support Order**

   All states have official child support guidelines. The guidelines are used to calculate how much a parent should contribute to financially support his or her child.

   Your child support office will be able to tell you how support amounts are set in your state and can request medical support for your child.

3. Enforce The Child Support Order

The most successful way to collect child support is by direct withholding from the obligated parent's paycheck. Most child support orders require the employer to withhold the money that is ordered for child support, and send it to the state child support office. Your child support office can tell you about this procedure.

At any of these steps, the child support office may need to know where the noncustodial parent lives or where he or she works. When a parent's whereabouts are not known, it is usually possible for the child support office to find him or her with the help of state agencies, such as the Department of Motor Vehicles, or the Federal Parent Locator Service. Your caseworker can tell you what information is needed to find an absent parent or the employer.

There are several ways Administration for Childrens and Families (ACF) collects and enforces child support:

- Withhold income
- Deny Passports
- Intercept federal payments
- Set liens on property
- Withhold tax refunds
- Report child support debts to credit bureaus
- Suspend or revoke drivers, professional, occupational, and recreational licenses

How And Where Do I Apply?

Contact your local child support office to apply for child support services. Your state may allow you to apply online.

Here are some things you might need to provide. Ask your local office for a complete list.

- Information about the noncustodial parent
- Birth certificates of children
- If paternity is an issue, written statements (letters or notes) in which the alleged father has said or implied that he is the father of the child
- Your child support order, divorce decree, or separation agreement if you have one
- Records of any child support received in the past

- Information about your income and assets

- Information about expenses, such as your child's healthcare, daycare, or special needs

What Does The Child Support Program Do?

State and tribal child support programs locate noncustodial parents, establish paternity, establish and enforce support orders, modify orders when appropriate, collect and distribute child support payments, and refer parents to other services. While programs vary from state to state, their services are available to all parents who need them.

The program's mission is to increase parental support of children by:

- Locating parents

- Establishing legal fatherhood (paternity)

- Establishing and enforcing fair support orders

- Increasing healthcare coverage for children

- Referring parents to employment services, helping to build healthy family relationships, supporting responsible fatherhood and helping to prevent and reduce family violence

---

The Children's Father Lost His Job And Is Collecting Unemployment Compensation. Can Child Support Payments Be Deducted And Sent To Me?

Yes. Unemployment compensation, and other state and Federal benefits can be tapped for child support. Ask your caseworker about the procedures, and make sure you tell your caseworker immediately if you learn about changes in the father's employment situation.

(*Source: "Handbook On Child Support Enforcement," publications.usa.gov.*)

What Are The Roles Of The State And Federal Child Support Programs?

State, tribal and local child support offices provide day to day operation of the program. They manage the child support caseload.

The federal role is to provide funding, issue policy, ensure that federal requirements are met, and interact with other federal agencies that help support the child support program.

Chapter 68
Teen Fatherhood Rights And Responsibilities

Finding out that you are going to be a father will probably generate mixed feelings, ranging from shock and uncertainty to acceptance and excitement. While facing parenthood can be challenging at any age, it is particularly difficult for teenagers, since you must take responsibility for a new life before you have reached full maturity yourself. Having a child is a serious, lifelong commitment that you may not feel ready to take on. But it may help to know that you are not alone. Around 750,000 teenaged girls become pregnant in the United States every year, so an equal number of young men learn that they are going to be fathers.

Even as a teenager, becoming a father involves legal rights and responsibilities. Although the laws vary by state, it is important to understand and exercise your rights, as well as to accept and meet your responsibilities. Ideally, you will be able to maintain a good relationship with the young woman carrying the baby, even if she is no longer your partner. This is the easiest way to ensure that you can play an active role in your child's life. But even if you do not have a good relationship with the mother, you can still love and support your child.

Rights Of Teen Fathers

All fathers, regardless of their age, have rights with regard to their children. If you are a young, unmarried father, it may be a bit more complicated to claim your parental rights than it would be for an adult who is married to the baby's mother. Here is a rundown of some of the basic rights available to fathers in most states:

- **The right to establish paternity**

  The first step in exercising your parental rights is to be legally recognized as the child's father. Although married fathers do not need to establish paternity, unmarried fathers

"Teen Fatherhood Rights And Responsibilities," © 2017 Omnigraphics. Reviewed March 2017.

usually must confirm their status through a DNA test performed after the baby's birth. In some states, you may be able to do it by signing a legal document known as an Acknowledgment of Paternity. Once you have legal standing as the father, you have the right to be involved in the child's life.

- **The right to have a say in pregnancy decisions**

  Most states require pregnant teens under age 18 to notify their parents or obtain parental consent before terminating a pregnancy. The decision of whether to continue a pregnancy ultimately belongs to the woman, though, and the father does not have a legal right to participate in it. However, most states require the consent of both biological parents before a child can be placed for adoption. Since some states do not make much effort to identify, locate, and notify unmarried birth fathers, it is important to establish paternity and keep the lines of communication open with the birth mother to ensure that your parental rights are protected.

- **The right to custody**

  If a child's parents are unmarried, most states will award sole physical custody to the biological mother unless the biological father petitions a court for joint or shared custody. This means that the child will most likely live with the mother unless you establish paternity and convince a judge that spending part of the time with you is in the child's best interest. In most cases, though, the court will award joint legal custody, which allows both parents to participate equally in decisions affecting the child's health, education, and welfare. Legal custody also gives you the right to access the child's medical records and school information.

- **The right to visitation**

  As a father, you have a right to get to know your child and be present in your child's life. Even if the child lives with the mother full time, you are entitled to visit the child according to a regular schedule that is approved by a family court judge. A typical visitation schedule might allow you to see your child one night per week and every other weekend. You may need to take legal action to ensure that you receive your visitation rights.

Responsibilities Of Teen Fathers

Along with the rights of fatherhood come many responsibilities. For instance, you are responsible for supporting your child financially, ensuring that your child is safe and well cared for, and making decisions that are in your child's best interest. Here is a rundown of some of the basic responsibilities of fathers in most states:

- **The responsibility to provide financial support**

  If the child's mother is awarded sole physical custody, you will probably be required to make child support payments to help cover the child's living expenses. The amount varies depending on state laws and the respective income of each parent. Child support helps pay for such expenses as food, clothing, education, daycare, and healthcare. Failure to pay court-ordered child support can result in such penalties as fines, withheld wages, suspension of a driver's license or passport, arrest, and imprisonment.

- **The responsibility to be involved in parenting**

  Studies have shown that active, involved fathers have a positive impact on a child's development. When children bond with their father, sons show fewer behavioral problems and daughters show fewer emotional problems. You can provide love and support by spending time with your child and helping with child care. Although dealing with an infant may seem overwhelming, it is important to form a bond at this early stage by learning to feed your baby, change diapers, and use a car seat properly. Attending a parenting class may help you feel more comfortable with these responsibilities.

- **The responsibility to be a good role model**

  Once you become a father, your child needs to become your main focus. Rather than partying, dating, or experimenting with alcohol or drugs, you should devote most of your energy to spending time with your child and providing a stable environment for your child's growth. An important part of building a solid future for your child is getting a good education. You should be sure to get your high school diploma and pursue grants, loans, and work-study opportunities to go to college. Pursuing an education will not only make you better equipped to provide for your child, but will also provide a good example for your child to follow.

Although the responsibilities of being a father may seem overwhelming, there are plenty of sources of help available. Your parents, family members, friends, school counselor, or medical provider should be able to provide you with advice and assistance as you learn about fatherhood.

References

1. "Becoming a Father," Young Men's Health, 2017.
2. Derr, Mary Krane. "Father's Rights in Teen Pregnancy," Livestrong, October 6, 2015.

3. Hardcastle, Mike. "Teen Fatherhood: Rights and Responsibilities of Being a Teen Dad," About Relationships, May 5, 2016.

4. Julia, Brooke. "How to Be a Teenage Father," How to Adult, 2017.

Part Eight
If You Need More Information

Chapter 69

Directory Of Teen Pregnancy Resources

Information About Sexual Health, Pregnancy, And Birth

Administration for Children and Families (ACF)

U.S. Department of Health and Human Services (HHS)
370 L'Enfant Promenade S.W.
Washington, DC 20447
Phone: 202-401-9333
Fax: 202-690-7441
Website: www.acf.hhs.gov

Advocates for Youth

2000 M St. N.W., Ste. 750
Washington, DC 20036
Phone: 202-419-3420
Fax: 202-419-1448
Website: www.advocatesforyouth.org

American College of Nurse-Midwives (ACNM)

8403 Colesville Rd., Ste. 1550
Silver Spring, MD 20910
Phone: 240-485-1800
Fax: 240-485-1818
Website: www.midwife.org

Resources in this chapter were compiled from several sources deemed reliable; all contact information was verified and updated in March 2017.

American College of Obstetricians and Gynecologists (ACOG)
409 12th St. S.W.
Washington, DC 20090-6920
Toll-Free: 800-673-8444
Phone: 202-638-5577
Website: www.acog.org
E-mail: resources@acog.org

American Pregnancy Association
3007 Skyway Cir. N., Ste. 800
Irving, TX 75038
Toll-Free: 800-672-2296
Phone: 972-550-0140
Website: www.americanpregnancy.org
E-mail: info@americanpregnancy.org

American Social Health Association (ASHA)
P.O. Box 13827
Research Triangle Park, NC 27709
Phone: 919-361-8400
Fax: 919-361-8425
Website: www.ashastd.org
E-mail: info@ashastd.org

Black Women's Health Imperative
(Formerly known as National Black Women's Health Project)
55 M St. N.W., Ste. 940
Washington, DC 20003
Phone: 202-548-4000
Website: www.blackwomenshealth.org
E-mail: imperative@bwhi.org

Child Care Aware of America (CCAO)
1515 N. Courthouse Rd.
Second Fl.
Arlington, VA 22201
Toll-Free: 800-424-2246
Phone: 703-341-4100
Fax: 703-341-4101
Toll-Free TTY: 866-278-9428
Website: www.childcareaware.org
E-mail: info@childcareaware.org

Child Welfare Information Gateway

Children's Bureau/ACYF
330 C St. S.W.
Washington, DC 20201
Toll-Free: 800-394-3366
Phone: 703-385-7565
Fax: 703-385-3206
Website: www.childwelfare.gov
E-mail: info@childwelfare.gov

Childbirth Connection

National Partnership for Women & Families
1875 Connecticut Ave. N.W.
Ste. 650
Washington, DC 20009
Phone: 202-986-2600
Fax: 202-986-2539
Website: www.childbirthconnection.org
E-mail: info@nationalpartnership.org

Eunice Kennedy Shriver National Institute of Child Health and Human Development (NICHD)

Information Resource Center
P.O. Box 3006
Rockville, MD 20847
Toll-Free: 800-370-2943
Fax: 866-760-5947
Toll-Free TTY: 888-320-6942
Website: www.nichd.nih.gov
E-mail: NICHDInformationResourceCenter@mail.nih.gov

Focus Adolescent Services

1113 Woodland Rd.
Ste.1000
Salisbury, MD 21801
Phone: 443-358-4691
Website: www.focusas.org

Guttmacher Institute

125 Maiden Ln.
Seventh Fl.
New York, NY 10038
Toll-Free: 800-355-0244
Phone: 212-248-1111
Fax: 212-248-1951
Website: www.guttmacher.org

Health Resources and Services Administration (HRSA)

Maternal and Child Health HRSA Information Center
P.O. Box 2910
Merrifield, VA 22116
Toll-Free Fax: 888-ASK-HRSA (888-275-4772)
Toll-Free TTY: 877-4TY-HRSA (877-489-4772)
Website: mchb.hrsa.gov
E-mail: ask@hrsa.gov

Lamaze International

2025 M St. N.W., Ste. 800
Washington, DC 20036-3309
Toll-Free: 800-368-4404
Phone: 202-367-1128
Fax: 202-367-2128
Website: www.lamaze.org
E-mail: info@lamaze.org

March of Dimes

Pregnancy and Newborn Health Service Center
1275 Mamaroneck Ave.
White Plains, NY 10605
Phone: 914-997-4488
Website: www.marchofdimes.com/pnhec/pnhec.asp

The National Campaign to Prevent Teen and Unplanned Pregnancy

1776 Massachusetts Ave. N.W., Ste. 200
Washington, DC 20036
Phone: 202-478-8500
Fax: 202-478-8588
Website: www.teenpregnancy.org
E-mail: campaign@teenpregnancy.org

National Domestic Violence Hotline

P.O. Box 161810
Austin, TX 78716
Toll-Free: 800-799-SAFE (800-799-7233)
Phone: 512-794-1133
Toll-Free TTY: 800-787-3224
Website: www.thehotline.org

National Sexual Assault Hotline

Toll-Free Fax: 800-656-HOPE (800-656-4673)
Website: www.rainn.org/about-national-sexual-assault-telephone-hotline

Planned Parenthood Federation of America

123 William St.
10th Fl.
New York, NY 10038
Toll-Free: 800-430-4907
Phone: 212-541-7800
Fax: 212-245-1845
Website: www.plannedparenthood.org
E-mail: info@ppau.org

Preeclampsia Foundation

6905 N. Wickham Rd.
Ste. 302
Melbourne, FL 32940
Toll-Free: 800-665-9341
Phone: 321-421-6957
Fax: 321-821-0450
Website: www.preeclampsia.org
E-mail: info@preeclampsia.org

Sexuality Information and Education Council of the United States (SIECUS)

1012 14th St. N.W., Ste. 1108
Washington, DC 20005
Phone: 202-265-2405
Fax: 202-462-2340
Website: www.siecus.org
E-mail: siecus@siecus.org

Womenshealth.gov

U.S. Department of Health and Human Services (HHS)
8270 Willow Oaks Corporate Dr.
Ste. 101
Fairfax, VA 22031
Toll-Free: 800-994-9662
Phone: 202-690-7650
Fax: 202-205-2631
Website: www.womenshealth.gov/Pregnancy

Breastfeeding And Postpartum Support

International Lactation Consultant Association (ILCA)

110 Horizon Dr.
Ste. 210
Raleigh, NC 27615
Toll-Free: 888-ILCA-IS-U (888-452-2478)
Phone: 919-861-5577
Fax: 919-459-2075
Website: www.ilca.org
E-mail: info@ilca.org

La Leche League International (LLLI)

110 Horizon Dr.
Ste. 210
Raleigh, NC 27615
Toll-Free: 877-4LA LECHE (877-452-5324)
Phone: 919-459-2167
Fax: 919-459-2075
Toll-Free Fax: 800-LALECHE (800-525-3243)
Website: www.lalecheleague.org
E-mail: info@llli.org

Nursing Mothers Counsel (NMC)

P.O. Box 5024
San Mateo, CA 94402-0024
Phone: 650-327-MILK (650-327-6455)
Website: www.nursingmothers.org
E-mail: info@nursingmothers.org

Postpartum Education for Parents (PEP)

P.O. Box 261
Santa Barbara, CA 93116
Phone: 805-564-3888 (24–hour service)
Website: www.sbpep.org
E-mail: pepboard@sbpep.org

Chapter 70

Directory Of Assistance Resources For Low-Income Pregnant Women

America's Essential Hospitals
401 Ninth St. N.W., Ste. 900
Washington, DC 20004
Phone: 202-585-0100
Fax: 202-585-0101
Website: essentialhospitals.org
E-mail: info@essentialhospitals.org

American Public Human Services Association (APHSA)
1133 19th St. N.W.
Ste. 400
Washington, DC 20036
Phone: 202-682-0100
Fax: 202-289-6555
Website: www.aphsa.org

Center for Health Care Strategies, Inc. (CHCS)
200 American Metro Blvd.
Ste. 119
Hamilton, NJ 08619
Phone: 609-528-8400
Fax: 609-586-3679
Website: www.chcs.org

Resources in this chapter were compiled from several sources deemed reliable; all contact information was verified and updated in March 2017.

Centers for Medicare and Medicaid Services (CMS)

7500 Security Blvd.
Baltimore, MD 21244-1850
Toll-Free: 877-267-2323
Phone: 410-786-3000
TTY: 410-786-0727
Toll-Free TTY: 866-226-1819
Website: www.cms.gov

Federal Office of Rural Health Policy (FORHP)

Health Resources and Services Administration (HRSA)
5600 Fishers Ln.
10B-45
Rockville, MD 20857
Phone: 301-443-0835
Fax: 301-443-2803
Website: www.hrsa.gov/ruralhealth
E-mail: ruralpolicy@hrsa.gov

National Academy for State Health Policy (NASHP)

10 Free St.
Second Fl.
Portland, ME 04101
Phone: 207-874-6524
Fax: 207-874-6527
Website: www.nashp.org
E-mail: info@nashp.org

National Advocates for Pregnant Women (NAPW)

15 W. 36th St., Ste. 901
New York, NY 10018-7910
Phone: 212-255-9252
Fax: 212-255-9253
Website: advocatesforpregnantwomen.org
E-mail: info@advocatesforpregnantwomen.org

National Coalition on Health Care (NCHC)

1111 14th St. N.W., Ste. 900
Washington, DC 20005
Phone: 202-638-7151
Fax: 202-638-7166
Website: www.nchc.org

National Health Law Program (NHelp)

3701 Wilshire Blvd., Ste. 750
Los Angeles, CA 90010
Phone: 310-204-6010
Fax: 310-368-0774
Website: www.healthlaw.org
E-mail: nhelp@healthlaw.org

National Rural Health Association (NRHA)

4501 College Blvd.
Ste. 225
Leawood, KS 66211-1921
Phone: 816-756-3140
Fax: 816-756-3144
Website: www.ruralhealthweb.org

Robert Wood Johnson Foundation (RWJF)

50 College Rd. E.
Princeton, NJ 08540-6614
Toll-Free: 877-843-RWJF (877-843-7953)
Website: www.rwjf.org

Second Chance Homes

U.S. Department of Housing and Urban Development (HUD)
451 Seventh St. S.W.
Washington, DC 20410
Phone: 202-708-1112
TTY: 202-708-1455
Website: portal.hud.gov/hudportal/HUD?src=/program_offices/public_indian_housing/other/sch

Special Supplemental Nutrition Program for Women, Infants, and Children (WIC)

Food and Nutrition Service (FNS), U.S. Department of Agriculture (USDA)
3101 Park Center Dr.
Rm. 520
Alexandria, VA 22302
Phone: 703-305-2062
Fax: 703-305-2196
Website: www.fns.usda.gov/wic/women-infants-and-children-wic
E-mail: wichq-web@fns.usda.gov

Urban Institute
2100 M St. N.W.
Washington, DC 20037
Phone: 202-833-7200
Website: www.urban.org

Chapter 71

Directory Of Education Resources For Teen Parents

Education Resources

American Council on Education (ACE)
One Dupont Cir. N.W.
Washington, DC 20036-1193
Phone: 202-939-9300
Website: www.acenet.edu

Job Corps
U.S. Department of Labor (DOL)
200 Constitution Ave. N.W.
Ste. N4463
Washington, DC 20210
Toll-Free: 800-773-JOBS (800-773-5627)
Phone: 202-693-3000
Fax: 202-693-2767
TTY: 877-889-5627
Website: jobcorps.dol.gov
E-mail: national_office@jobcorps.gov

Resources in this chapter were compiled from several sources deemed reliable; all contact information was verified and updated in March 2017.

U.S. Department of Education (ED)

400 Maryland Ave. S.W.
Washington, DC 20202
Toll-Free: 800-USA-LEARN (800-872-5327)
Phone: 202-401-2000
Fax: 202-401-0689
TTY: 800-437-0833
Website: www.ed.gov

Online Directories For State-Specific Help

American Association Of Community Colleges

An advocacy organization for the nation's community colleges that represents nearly 1,200 two-year, associate degree–granting institutions.
Website: www.aacc.nche.edu/Pages/default.aspx

State Coordinators For The Education Of Children And Youth Experiencing Homelessness

This document provides the list of State Coordinators who are responsible for ensuring the continued education of youth who are experiencing homelessness.
Website: eclkc.ohs.acf.hhs.gov/hslc/tta-system/family/family/Homelessness/StateCoordinator.htm

State Director Of Adult Education

This webpage offers contact information of department of education, the higher education agency, special education agency and adult education agency in your state.
Website: www2.ed.gov/about/contacts/state/index.html

State Tech Prep Coordinator

This webpage contains the contact information of State Tech Prep Coordinators.
Website: techedmagazine.com/node/4145

Financial Aid Information For Postsecondary Education

College Board Scholarship Search

National Office
45 Columbus Ave.
New York, NY 10023-6917
Toll-Free: 866-630-9305
Phone: 212-713-8000
Website: bigfuture.collegeboard.org/scholarship-search

FastWeb

FastWeb, LLC
444 N. Michigan Ave., Ste. 600
Chicago, IL 60611
Website: www.fastweb.com
E-mail: info@fastweb.com

Federal Student Aid

Toll-Free: 800-4-FED-AID (800-433-3243)
Phone: 319-337-5665
TTY/TDD: 800-730-8913
Website: studentaid.ed.gov

FinAid

FinAid Page, LLC
P.O. Box 2056
Cranberry Township, PA 16066-1056
Phone: 724-538-4500
Fax: 724-538-4502
Website: www.finaid.org
E-mail: questions@finaid.org

Free Application for Federal Student Aid (FAFSA)

Toll-Free: 800-4-FED-AID (800-433-3243)
Phone: 319-337-5665
TTY/TDD: 800-730-8913
Website: www.fafsa.ed.gov

National Association of Student Financial Aid Administrators (NASFAA)

1101 Connecticut Ave. N.W.
Ste. 1100
Washington, DC 20036-4303
Phone: 202-785-0453
Fax: 202-785-1487
Website: www.nasfaa.org

Sallie Mae Bank

P.O. Box 3319
Wilmington, DE 19804-4319
Toll-Free: 855-SLM-LOAN (855-756-5626)
Phone: 317-570-7397
Toll-Free Fax: 800-848-1949
TDD: 888-TDD-SLMA (888-833-7562)
Website: www.salliemae.com

Index

Index

Page numbers that appear in *Italics* refer to tables or illustrations. Page numbers that have a small 'n' after the page number refer to citation information shown as Notes. Page numbers that appear in **Bold** refer to information contained in boxes within the chapters.

A

abdominal pain
    eclampsia 225
    iron deficiency anemia 218
    miscarriage 261
abortion
    miscarriage 261
    overview 57–61
    parenting options 69
"Abortion" (Planned Parenthood Federation of America Inc.) 57n
abortion pill, effectiveness 58
"About Second Chance Homes" (HUD) 353n
abstinence
    birth control, tabulated *29*
    Family Youth Service Bureau (FYSB) **5**
    teen pregnancy 19
abuse
    depression 132
    emancipation 346
    overview 11–5
    preterm labor 233
    see also domestic violence
accreditation, child care providers 370
acetylsalicylate (aspirin) 143
ACF *see* Administration for Childrens and Families
ACF/FYSB prevention programs **5**

acquired immune deficiency syndrome (AIDS), high-risk pregnancy 192
Administration for Children and Families (ACF)
    contact 391
    publication, child support 381n
adolescent childbearing 5
adoptions
    emancipation 345
    fatherhood 386
    overview 63–8
    paternity 69
Advocates for Youth, contact 391
aerobic activity
    physical activity 112
    prenatal care 88
    weight gain during pregnancy 121
Affordable Care Act
    low-cost birth control 37
    teen pregnancy prevention 5, 20
afterbirth 298
age factor
    births and birth rates 9
    smoking **165**, **167**
AIDS *see* acquired immune deficiency syndrome
alcohol
    abuse and pregnancy 12
    emancipation *345*

409

P